EAT
YOUR
WAY
TO A
SIX PACK

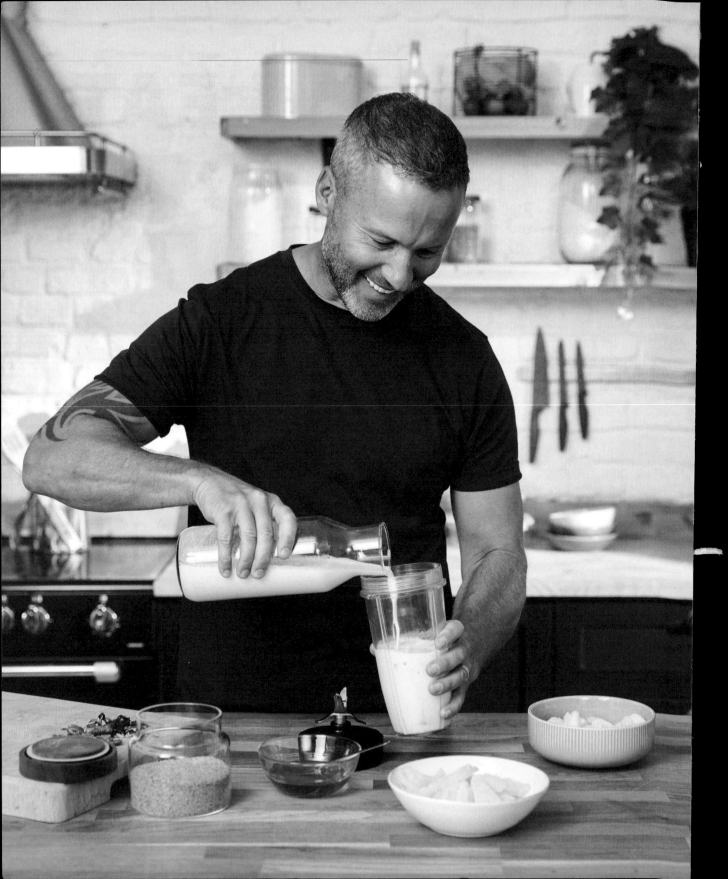

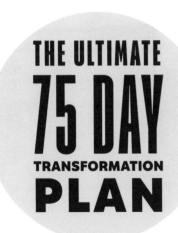

THE ULTIMATE
75 DAY
TRANSFORMATION
PLAN

EAT YOUR WAY TO A SIX PACK

SCOTT HARRISON

Photography by David Cummings

CONTENTS

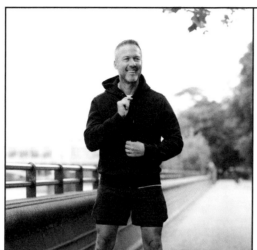

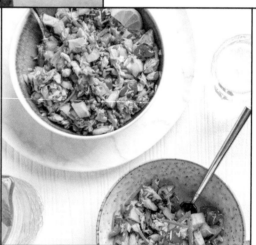

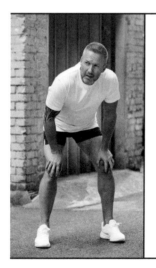

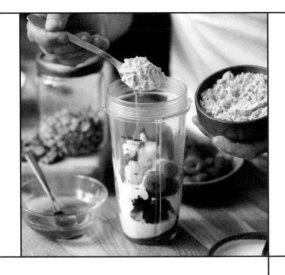

KNOW YOUR NUTRITION

TRANSFORM BODY AND MIND

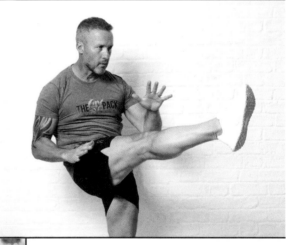

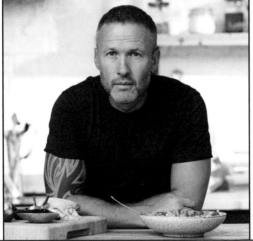

THE SIX PACK EXPERTS

HEY FRIENDS . . .

Welcome! By picking up my book, *Eat Your Way to a Six Pack*, you've taken the first crucial step toward a life-changing journey. I commend your commitment to transforming not only your relationship with food and drink but also your relationship with yourself. I'm sure you are here because you want to feel stronger, more confident, and amazing, and I'm here to help you achieve this.

It's important that you know that my journey started just like yours. I realized that I needed to make some clear changes in my life, which included the way I used food for comfort, my approach to alcohol, and how my eating habits led to poor health and excess weight. I had slipped away from looking after ME. I needed to reset my mind, focus on an end goal, and use mindfulness and positivity to transform myself!

When I started on my health journey, I leaned heavily on my passion for cooking and learned to create recipes that were balanced, healthy, and tasty, which I wanted to return to again and again. Martial arts taught me the invaluable lessons of focus, mindfulness, and positivity, and these became instrumental in not just setting goals but achieving them.

As my body started to respond to a healthy diet and physical training, I shared my experiences on social media, and the response was astounding. People were inspired by my results and even began to join in. My followers grew, and the culmination of these experiences led to the creation of something truly magical—The Six Pack Revolution.

Today, I stand as living proof that this transformative program truly works. I am a testament to the power of dedication—my life is filled with fitness, happiness, abundance, and optimal health. So, my mission now is simple. I want to share my knowledge and positivity with you and to support you through your own journey toward health and well-being.

Whether you follow a plant-based lifestyle or not, my book provides a roadmap for success. Within its pages, you'll discover a collection of carefully crafted recipes that are both delicious and healthy, offering nourishment for every palate. By adhering to the principles outlined in this book and putting in the hard work, you will experience a complete rebalancing of both body and mind. However, remember, that this is about more than just physical changes. It's a holistic transformation that encompasses your entire being.

Writing this book has been another milestone on my health and wellness journey, and I'm grateful for the opportunity to connect with you as you embark on this path. Know that I am here to guide, motivate, and uplift you, every step of the way.

Keep an eye out for my upcoming projects as I continue to strive for balanced nutrition and exercise for all. Until we meet again, good luck on becoming the best version of yourself.

YOU'VE GOT THIS!

YOUR TRANSFORMATIONS

All these results were achieved in just 75 days.

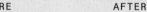

Ellie Small

"Wow! What can I say? The Six Pack Revolution does what it says on the package! It gave me a new way of looking at food... and who would have thought that you could eat six tasty meals a day and get amazing results?! I have loads of allergies and found that the simplicity of swapping one ingredient for another really worked. The support and community also makes being on the plan really enjoyable."

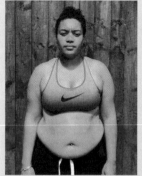
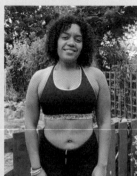

Claire Sipple

"I know it's a clichéd thing to say, but The Six Pack Revolution literally changed my life. As well as the obvious weight loss, it rewired my relationship with food and nutrition. No longer do I have anxiety attacks, and, even though I'm currently navigating menopause, I feel so in control of my health and well-being."

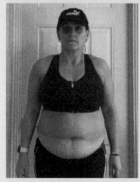
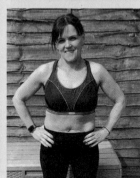

Matthew Jenkinson

"I was blown away by the results I achieved, not just physically but also mentally. What really surprised me was how delicious the meal plans are and the variety of workouts, most of which can be done at home. The team support you receive is also incredible. I'd highly recommend this to anyone looking to get in shape, improve their fitness, or boost their mental well-being. Thanks again, 'team.'"

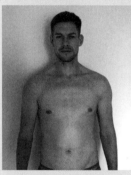
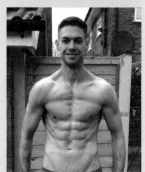

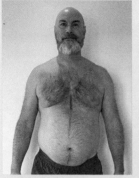 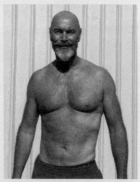

Paul Williams

"The Six Pack Revolution is a life-changing program that helped me transform my physical appearance—I lost a total of 37.5lb in 75 days! The knowledgeable trainers and nutritionists led me through demanding yet rewarding workouts, pushing me well past my comfort zone by inspiring and encouraging me. The nutritionally sound plan made sure I received the necessary fuel to train, while also improving my dietary habits."

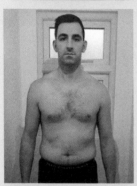 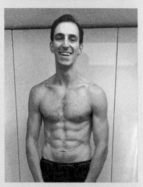

Richard Servidei

"The Six Pack Revolution has given me more than just a physical transformation. With exceptional support, I completed the Signature wave and became stronger, not only in body but also in mind, with a newfound belief in my own potential. This plan has forever changed my life by removing barriers of self-doubt, giving me clarity of thought and resilience, while reminding me to embrace each and every day. I am grateful to Scott and the team for the impact it has had on my life."

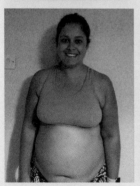 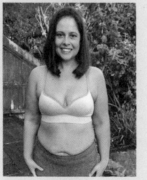

Caron Pollard

"The Six Pack Revolution has empowered me to reclaim my identity as a woman and business owner and feel confident about how I show up in different areas of my life —who is this woman?! The program has enabled me to undo a lot of damage from living with lymphedema and lipedema and has vastly improved my condition when I thought there was no hope. I am forever grateful for this newfound ability to make powerful choices, which will have long-term benefits for me and my family."

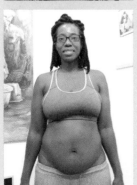 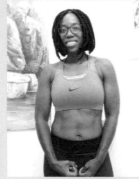

Nana Tamakloe

"The Six Pack Revolution program is amazing. Why? It is not just about weight loss and healthy living, but it taps into the inner recesses of the mind to connect it with the body and soul, achieving great heights in mental and physical fitness. The result of SPR has been distinct Self-Mastery. What is more life-changing than that?"

Edward Nascimento

"The Six Pack Revolution completely changed my life! If I'm honest, I was so skeptical before joining, and the reason was because I'd tried so many diets, and joined the gym countless ti,mes too, but never really achieved anything. But wow, what can I say—the results speak for themselves. If you follow the program, you will get the results and, best of all, you are going to feel great! At last, I found myself healthy again!"

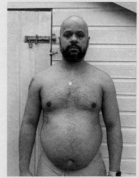 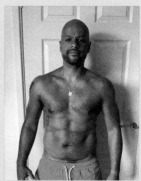

Louise Stevens

"The Six Pack Revolution really helped me regain my body confidence after having my daughter. As any new mom will tell you, those first few months are extremely tough, and I definitely felt like I'd lost who I was as an individual. Therefore, six months postpartum, I decided to join. SPR reset my relationship with food and taught me that there's always time to exercise, no matter what! By the time I'd completed my 75 days, I was fitter, stronger, and healthier than before my pregnancy, even pre-COVID, and dropped two dress sizes in the process."

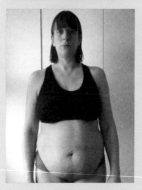 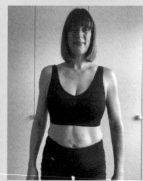

Patrick Bennett

"For years, I struggled to manage that middle-age spread. I tried exercising with some careful food choices, but nothing changed. With The Six Pack Revolution, my shape, weight, and how I looked completely changed. I felt healthier, lighter, and fitter, and my middle-age spread was gone. Thank you, SPR, for the magic and for showing me a much healthier lifestyle."

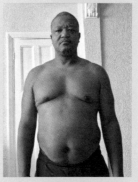 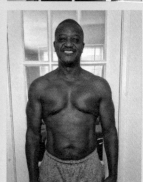

Lisa Hord

"I was skeptical, but this absolutely works and has changed my life for the better. I've been overweight for most of my life, and this is the fittest and healthiest I have ever felt!"

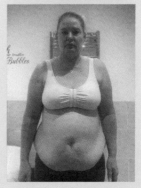 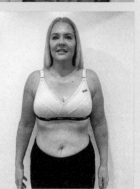

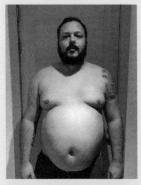 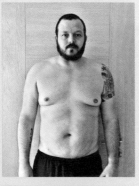

Ben Cassar

"You might have heard it a lot already, but The Six Pack Revolution is truly a life-changing experience in a holistic way. I was 298lb before I started the diet. I suffered from back pain, high blood pressure, kidney stones, and, the worst of all, loss of mobility. But with the program, I regained the will to play, hike, and experience life with my kids! If you are thinking about SPR, please don't! JUST DO IT and experience the change yourself."

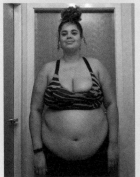 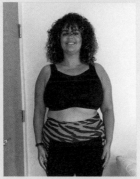

Laura Bartlett

"The Six Pack Revolution did what it said on the package. It revolutionized my life! Not only my body, but also my mind. Following the program was one of the best decisions I've made. Not only am I lighter and stronger, but I feel like the version of myself that has been missing is back in all of her glory. Except this time, I'm even better than ever."

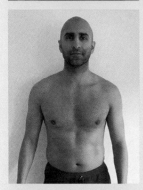 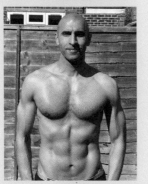

Imran Englfield

"After retiring from playing football for over 20 years, I found my weight increasing and mental health decreasing. The Six Pack Revolution not only saved me from a dark place but gave me amazing discipline in all aspects of my life. My transformation photo is simply a metaphor for how amazing I'm feeling in my mind."

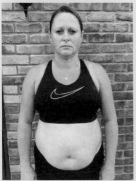 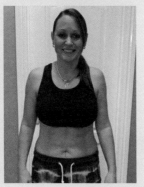

Angie Joyce

"I expected I would probably drop a dress size or two, but what I didn't expect was the profound feeling of happiness and clarity of mind. I am 50, yet have never felt better! I'll be forever grateful to Scotty and the team for showing me the key to health and happiness."

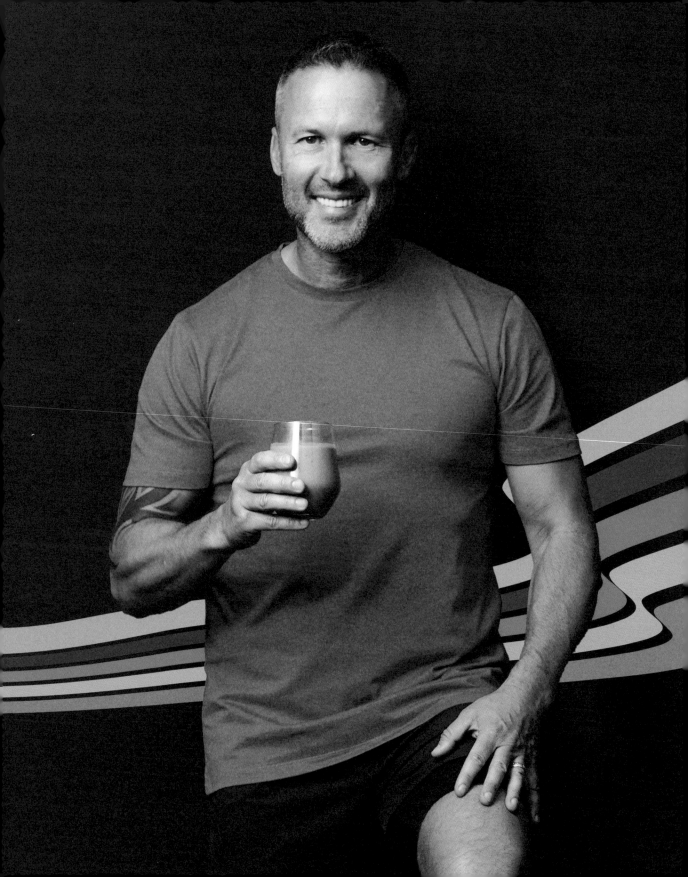

KNOW YOUR NUTRITION

Chapter One

MACRONUTRIENTS

 Let's delve into the powerhouse of nutrition—macronutrients! What are they, and what do they provide? These bad boys are the secret sauce behind a healthy body and mind, so pay close attention.

Macronutrients are the fundamental nutrients our bodies need in significant quantities in order to function and to thrive. They are the backbone of our energy levels, strength, and overall vitality. The three primary macronutrients are proteins, carbohydrates, and fats, and each plays a unique role in optimizing our health and fitness.

MICRONUTRIENTS—SMALL BUT MIGHTY

As we crush it with macronutrients, let's not forget the mini unsung heroes—micronutrients! These little champs, consisting of vitamins and minerals, are essential for keeping your body running like a well-oiled machine. From vitamin C, which boosts the immune system, to calcium that strengthens bones, these rock stars complement the work of macronutrients and deserve their share of the spotlight.

So, there you have it—the lowdown on micronutrients. Remember, it's all about balance and making small but smart choices every step of the way! Keep pushing forward, and let's make those dreams a reality!

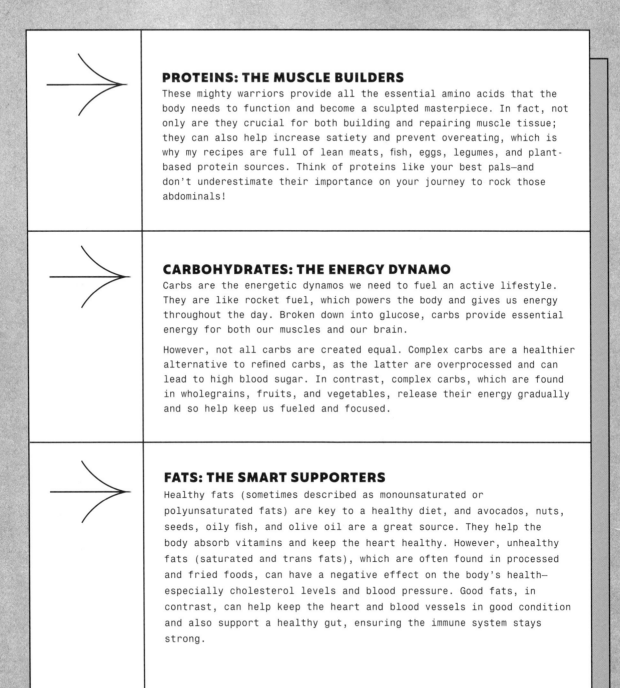

PROTEINS: THE MUSCLE BUILDERS

These mighty warriors provide all the essential amino acids that the body needs to function and become a sculpted masterpiece. In fact, not only are they crucial for both building and repairing muscle tissue; they can also help increase satiety and prevent overeating, which is why my recipes are full of lean meats, fish, eggs, legumes, and plant-based protein sources. Think of proteins like your best pals—and don't underestimate their importance on your journey to rock those abdominals!

CARBOHYDRATES: THE ENERGY DYNAMO

Carbs are the energetic dynamos we need to fuel an active lifestyle. They are like rocket fuel, which powers the body and gives us energy throughout the day. Broken down into glucose, carbs provide essential energy for both our muscles and our brain.

However, not all carbs are created equal. Complex carbs are a healthier alternative to refined carbs, as the latter are overprocessed and can lead to high blood sugar. In contrast, complex carbs, which are found in wholegrains, fruits, and vegetables, release their energy gradually and so help keep us fueled and focused.

FATS: THE SMART SUPPORTERS

Healthy fats (sometimes described as monounsaturated or polyunsaturated fats) are key to a healthy diet, and avocados, nuts, seeds, oily fish, and olive oil are a great source. They help the body absorb vitamins and keep the heart healthy. However, unhealthy fats (saturated and trans fats), which are often found in processed and fried foods, can have a negative effect on the body's health— especially cholesterol levels and blood pressure. Good fats, in contrast, can help keep the heart and blood vessels in good condition and also support a healthy gut, ensuring the immune system stays strong.

THE RULES

The Six Pack journey is centered around one key concept: balance. From nutrition and recipes to workouts and lifestyle, it provides the foundation for everything we do — achieving harmony is the key.

The Six Pack Revolution will show you how to use food in a positive way by giving you a routine of eating that keeps you feeling full, helps change the shape of your body, and boosts both your physical and mental health. You'll have more energy and more motivation, look incredible, and feel amazing!

IT'S SIMPLE: EAT SIX TIMES A DAY

Yes, six! That means three meals and three snacks from this book, each day. Or, the easiest and most popular way of following this program is to have two meals, two snacks, and two meal replacement smoothies/shakes a day. In addition, remember to refuel your muscles after your exercise challenges with one of our Post Workout Protein Smoothies (www.thesixpackrevolution.com/shop).

THE "LIKE FOR LIKE" RULE:

Every recipe can be tailored to your preferences

If there is an ingredient you are allergic to, or simply want to avoid, simply swap "like for like." The lean protein elements of each recipe can be switched for another lean protein source of the equivalent amount (easily facilitating vegan/vegetarian flexibility), but note that beef, pork, lamb, and duck are not part of the program. In the same way, any vegetable can be swapped for another, as long as you stick to the same quantity. And, if you'd rather have a teaspoon of olive oil on your salad instead of half an avocado (as per the recipe), then that's fine because you're swapping like for like... one source of healthy fats for another.

SIMPLE RULES OF THE HAND

This tailor-made approach uses your own hand size to measure your macronutrient intake at every meal. This ensures you are eating a balanced plate of food and keeps the process simple.

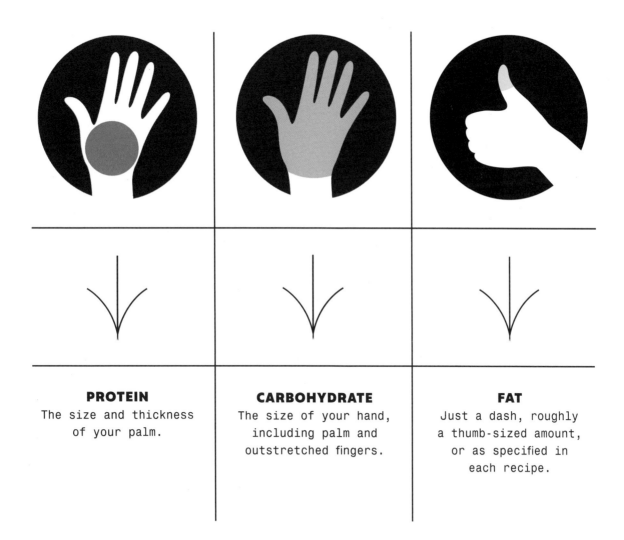

PROTEIN
The size and thickness of your palm.

CARBOHYDRATE
The size of your hand, including palm and outstretched fingers.

FAT
Just a dash, roughly a thumb-sized amount, or as specified in each recipe.

KEEPING HYDRATED: QUENCH YOUR THIRST

WATER—THE ELIXIR OF LIFE

Staying hydrated is more than just drinking enough water; it's a commitment to your well-being.

More than half of the human adult body is made of water, and it's essential for keeping the organs functioning properly, maintaining blood pressure, and helping the kidneys filter the blood and excrete toxins and waste. Plus, it lubricates joints, which is extra important when following a fitness regime.

Men should drink roughly 1 gallon of water per day, and women should drink roughly 3 quarts. When I wake up, I start my day with a large glass of water, and this should be your number-one priority too. If you're struggling to consume your daily amount, add a slice of lemon or other fruits, or you can drink it hot with a super-healthy organic green tea, which is proven to improve brain function.

By developing a healthy balance in your diet, you're empowering yourself to embrace a truly transformative lifestyle. Nourish your body with wholesome goodness, cultivate mindfulness in your eating habits, and embrace the power of healthy foods. Stay hydrated and witness the remarkable changes that unfold within you. Let's embark on this journey to lasting health, vitality, and happiness together!

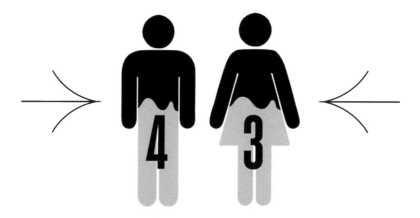

WHAT IS A 'SIX PACK'?

OK, WHAT IS A "SIX PACK," REALLY?

When I started on my health and fitness journey, a "six pack" represented my intention to build a strong and resilient body. I wanted the target of visible abdominal muscles so that I could see my progress with my own eyes as, with each step, I got closer to my goal. However, it soon became apparent that the term "six pack" could mean so much more than a physical manifestation. For me, it provided the foundation for personal growth, well-being, and a life of happiness and abundance. I now see a "six pack" as representing six core values, and I want to share these with you, as it's never too late to reshape your mindset with these vital values at its heart. Let's flip the script and reimagine what it means to develop a six pack of core values.

- **Empowerment and belief:** Think of it as the synchronicity between your physical prowess and mental fortitude, allowing you to conquer challenges with unwavering determination and a true belief in yourself. The Six Pack Revolution process will help you build confidence, not only in the physical sense but, even more importantly, mentally and emotionally too.

- **Strength and resilience:** Eating well, exercising, and simply taking caring of yourself cultivate resilience by fostering a mindset of consistent effort and gradual progress. In turn, this dedication and perseverance provides you with mental and emotional strength, which sustains you on your overall wellness journey.

- **Discipline and focus:** This is the cerebral equivalent of controlled repetitions. A healthy body and mind are nurtured by consistency in your thoughts, choices, and actions. Make sure that you constantly bring that mind of yours back to focusing on what you want instead of what you don't want.

- **Compassion and love:** Compassion is vital on your fitness journey, and the greatest love of all is to love yourself! Just as muscles require care, treating yourself kindly fosters a healthy relationship with your body. Extending this compassion to others, especially those close to you who share similar goals, helps build connections with others, which makes the process sustainable.

- **Gratitude and celebration:** Make sure you allow yourself to feel proud of all that you accomplish. Celebrating every small win will fuel your motivation, just as embracing gratitude for every step you make will breed a positive mindset and contribute to a successful and fulfilling life.

- **Authenticity and truth:** Just as physical balance ensures optimal body function, being real—aligning external effort with genuine internal values—creates a profound harmony. It's so much about embracing your unique path, believing in your purpose, working on your personal development, and sculpting a physique that mirrors your inner strength. Don't let anyone derail you from your mission toward a healthy and positive you!

I'm excited for you as you start on this life-changing journey. Remember, it's your evolution, not the endpoint, that is the goal. This will lead you to become the most genuine and vibrant you, for the rest of your wonderful life!

SIX IS THE MAGIC NUMBER

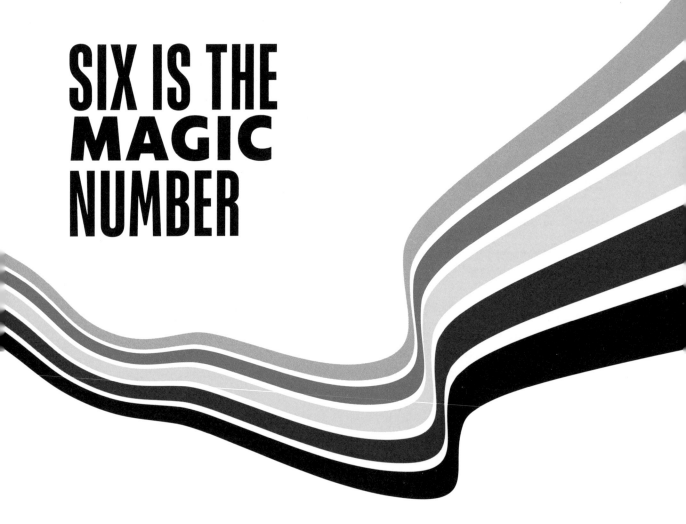

The Six Pack Revolution way means changing the way you eat. We believe in eating smaller portions, but more often. This means a combination of three balanced meals and three satisfying healthy snacks, which are designed to keep your body functioning optimally. Don't worry if it feels like you're eating more; here are all the reasons why you must trust the process and let the transformative magic unfold!

HERE'S THE <u>WHY</u> TO EATING 6 TIMES A DAY:

BOOSTING METABOLISM:

When you eat, your body uses energy to digest and process the food, known as the thermic effect of food (TEF). By eating more often, you increase the frequency of this process, which supports a healthy metabolism.

REGULATING BLOOD SUGAR LEVELS:

When you go for extended periods without eating, blood sugar can drop, leading to energy slumps and cravings for sugary or unhealthy foods. Frequent eating promotes a more consistent blood sugar level.

ENHANCED FAT BURNING:

When your body is provided with a steady stream of nutrients, it's less likely to store excess calories as fat. Additionally, regular eating helps maintain a consistent insulin response, which can also support a healthy metabolism.

ENHANCED SATIETY:

Eating more frequently can contribute to a greater feeling of fullness throughout the day. This heightened satiety helps reduce the desire to snack on unhealthy foods.

STABLE BLOOD PRESSURE:

Regular meals and snacks can help maintain stable blood pressure levels, contributing to heart health.

IMPROVED NUTRIENT DISTRIBUTION:

By spreading your meals and snacks, you ensure a more even distribution of essential nutrients over the course of the day.

STABLE MOOD AND MENTAL CLARITY:

Steady energy levels from frequent eating can positively influence your mood and feeling of mental clarity. This helps you maintain emotional well-being as well as focus and productivity.

BETTER DIGESTION AND GUT HEALTH:

Smaller, more frequent meals can ease the digestive burden on your system, enhancing overall gut health.

BALANCED HORMONAL RESPONSE:

Regular eating supports balanced hormone secretion, including those involved in appetite regulation, metabolism, and stress response.

PORTION CONTROL AND MINDFUL EATING:

With smaller, more frequent servings, you become more attuned to your body's hunger and satiety cues.

AN EXAMPLE OF A DAY IN THE LIFE OF THE SIX PACK REVOLUTION

This program is simple—you choose three meals and three snacks from the recipes in this book, which you can eat in any order throughout the day. However, try and keep a minimum of 2 hours and a maximum of 4 hours between eating, so plan your day accordingly.

The table below provides an example of a regular meal plan and a Meal Replacement food plan*.

The easiest and most popular way to do this program is to have two meals, two snacks, and two meal replacement smoothies/shakes a day and to always follow a workout with one of our Post Workout Protein Smoothies.

Our award-winning creamy, delicious Meal Replacement and Post Workout Protein Smoothies are made with the highest-quality ingredients and contain a whopping 30 servings in each pouch, making them one of the best values on the market. We also have our Overnight Oats and Sculpt Protein bars that can be used as your snack options.

This typical day is just an example—feel free to follow it as is or design your own food planner, if you are confident doing so. You can download a tracker here to make it a little easier for you. Visit **https://thesixpackrevolution.com/tracker**

8:00am

PROTEIN-PACKED BREAKFAST
Green Goddess Smoothie (p117)
OR *1 serving of The Six Pack Revolution Vanilla Caramel Heaven Meal Replacement Smoothie

10:30am

FUELING MID-MORNING
Feast from the East (p106)
OR *Thai Green Curry (p43)

12:30pm

NOURISHING LUNCH
Sweet and Sour (p89)
OR *1 serving of The Six Pack Revolution Decadent Chocolate Caramel Meal Replacement Smoothie

3:00pm

SATISFYING AFTERNOON SNACK
Strawberry Parfait (p160)
OR *Grilled Nectarines (p157)

6:30pm

WHOLESOME DINNER
Salmon and Goji Berry Curry (p38)
OR *Garlic and Chili Large Shrimp Singuine (p59)

9:00pm

LIGHT EVENING SNACK
Quinola (p122)
OR *The Six Pack Revolution Sculpt Bar

*An example of the MEAL REPLACEMENT FOOD PLAN

FLAVOR

No meal or snack should be naked—that's my mantra!

Eating with our senses is key: enticing culinary scents and vibrant colors on a plate make every meal something we can look forward to. No more beige—just pure, delicious, mouthwatering recipes that will keep us on plan and feeling fantastic!

FLAVOR HEROES

Here are some of my favorite herbs and spices. Try to include as many as you can in your meals, as they'll allow you to explore new tastes, plus they're full of micronutrients, polyphenols, and antioxidants, so they'll give you an extra boost of health at the same time.

- **Aromatic Garlic:** Besides its irresistible taste, garlic contains allicin, a compound known for its heart-protective properties, such as lowering cholesterol levels and supporting overall cardiovascular health.
- **Calming Cumin:** Full of beneficial compounds, cumin balances blood sugar levels, enhances overall well-being, and soothes away digestive discomfort. Its powerful anti-inflammatory effect earns it superfood status, in my opinion.
- **Earthy Turmeric:** Curcumin, the active compound in turmeric, is a powerful anti-inflammatory agent and antioxidant. It may also support joint health and help reduce chronic inflammation.
- **Exotic Ginger:** Gingerol, the bioactive compound in ginger, is known for its anti-nausea and anti-inflammatory properties, making it a popular remedy for digestive issues.
- **Fragrant Basil:** This herb is a great source of vitamins A, K, and C, as well as essential minerals, including potassium and calcium. It also contains flavonoids, which have many beneficial antioxidant properties.
- **Robust Rosemary:** Rosemary is rich in rosmarinic acid, a polyphenol with anti-inflammatory effects, which also enhances cognitive function and memory. Also high in antioxidants, rosemary provides good support for the immune system and can neutralize harmful free radicals.

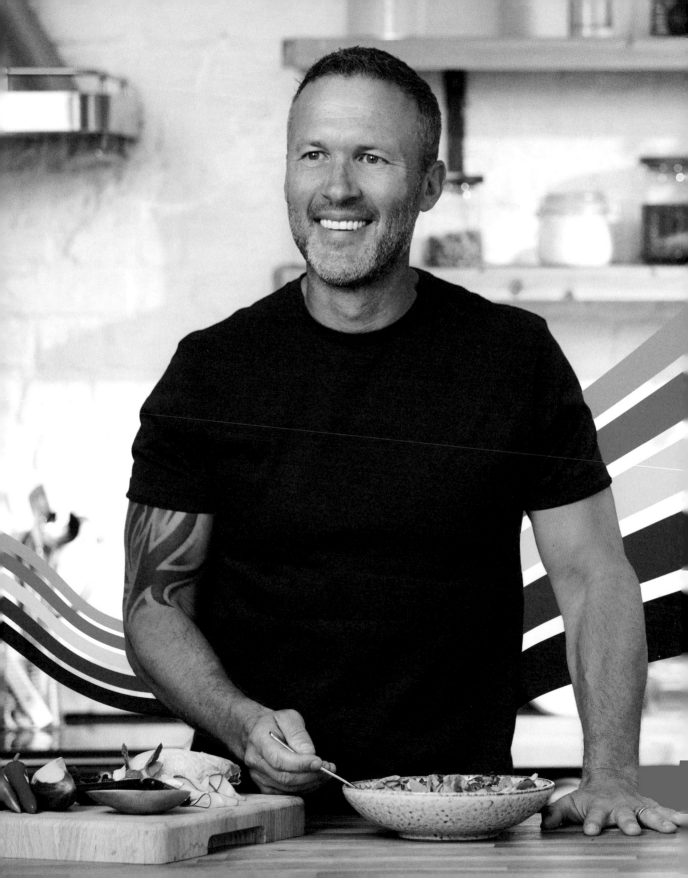

GET COOKING

Chapter Two

GETTING ORGANIZED

Getting organized in the kitchen is essential to your success, as it will enable you to create the delicious meals that will fuel your body and ensure you stay focused on the challenge ahead.

So, before delving into the culinary realm, let's set the stage by giving your home a refreshing sweep. Remove all the unhealthy and expired ingredients from your fridge and kitchen cupboards so you have space for your new kitchen companions.

There is very little equipment that you need to follow these recipes, and I'm sure you have most things already. However, the following items will certainly help you on your way, and the most important is the good-quality non-stick pan. My recipes deliberately use a certain amount of oil, so a good-quality non-stick pan is invaluable!

ESSENTIAL EQUIPMENT FOR YOUR KITCHEN CREATIONS:

- **Non-stick pan** – perfect for these recipes that use minimal oil
- **Set of quality knives** – for precise slicing and dicing
- **A few chopping boards** – ideally color-coded for different ingredients
- **Blender** – indispensable for smoothies, soups, sauces, and more
- **Spiralizer** – great for quickly transforming veggies into noodles

- **Mixing bowls, in assorted sizes**
- **Measuring tools** – measuring spoons, cups, jugs, and kitchen scales
- **Meal preparation containers** – in various sizes to store and portion out your creations
- **Freezer bags and ice cube trays** – to organize and preserve your ingredients and store leftovers and homemade sauces or stocks

TOP TIPS FOR COOKING SUCCESS

READ THE RECIPE

This may seem obvious, but trust me, it helps you feel well prepared. Before you start to cook, read through the entire recipe. Familiarize yourself with the steps and ingredients to avoid surprises along the way that can lead to failure.

PREP INGREDIENTS FIRST

Prepare all your ingredients before you start to cook so that you have everything ready and organized. This technique is known in the professional world as *mise en place*, and no self-respecting chef cooks any other way!

TASTE AS YOU GO

Don't be afraid to taste your dish as you cook, as it helps you adjust the seasonings and flavors to your liking and results in tastier food that enhances feelings of satiety.

THE "LIKE FOR LIKE" RULE

Remember this rule (p16), as it makes each recipe easily adaptable and provides you with almost endless variety. Good examples for swapping include turkey for tofu, chicken for high-protein meat alternative, salmon for seitan, white fish for beans, and so on. Vegetables and healthy fats can also be swapped for other equivalent kinds—just make sure you stick to the same quantity.

KEEP IT SIMPLE

Start with the simpler recipes and gradually build up your skills. As you gain confidence, you can tackle more complex dishes.

PLAN AHEAD

Planning your meals for the week is a game-changer. Take some time each week to plan your meals and your snacks, as preparation is key to staying on track!

BATCH COOKING IS THE SUPERHERO TECHNIQUE

Allocate a weekend to cook ahead, whip up extra portions of your favorite recipes, and freeze or refrigerate them for meals when you're short on time—your future self will be grateful. No more plan derailing!

Important: When batch cooking, doubling up on spices like chili, paprika, and other strong spices might result in an overly intense flavor or heat that could be too overwhelming when reheated. Spices tend to intensify as they sit, so it's advisable to start with a standard amount and adjust as you taste test or when you reheat individual portions.

ENJOY IT

Remember, cooking is an adventure, and it's okay to make mistakes. The most important thing is to enjoy the creative side of cooking and to build up your skills at your own pace. This way, you'll master the art of cooking and find joy in creating nourishing meals that contribute to your success on your health and fitness journey.

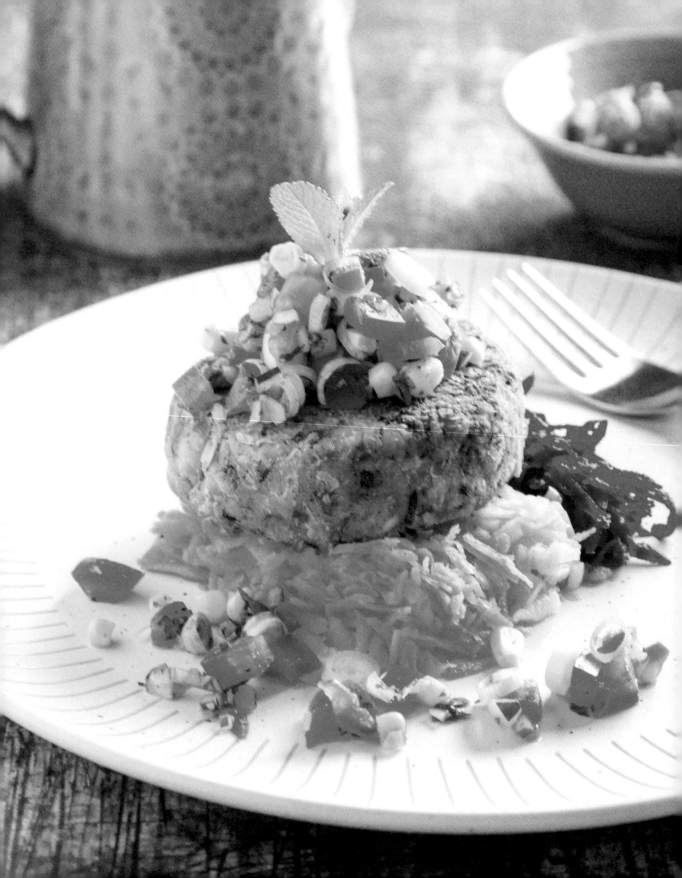

Here is a collection of my most-loved recipes, which I've designed to nourish you on every day of your transformation journey. Simply enjoy good food, and you'll start to feel the benefits right away.

MEALS

CRISPY BAKED TOFU

SERVES ONE

piece of firm tofu, 1½ x the size and thickness of your palm

zest of 1 lime

½ tsp white pepper

1 tsp mild curry powder

small handful of broccoli florets

5 shiitake mushrooms, sliced

2 tsp sesame seeds

small handful of bean sprouts

fresh cilantro leaves, to garnish

½ red chili, sliced

juice of ½ lime

Tofu is great for marinating and baking, as it absorbs all the flavor you can give it and turns golden around the edges. Bean sprouts are also full of vitamin C and calcium, and I love to eat them raw for that satisfying crunch.

1 Preheat the oven to 400°F and heat the broiler, adjusting the rack to the top half of the oven.

2 First, marinate the tofu. Place the tofu cubes in a mixing bowl with the lime zest, white pepper, and curry powder and mix well.

3 Transfer the marinated tofu to a baking sheet and broil for 5–10 minutes, turning regularly, until golden brown. Set aside.

4 Bring a pot of water to a boil and cook the broccoli for 1 minute, then drain and place in a bowl with the sliced mushroom and sesame seeds. Mix well.

5 Add the sesame-coated vegetables to the tray with the marinated tofu and cook in the oven for 5–10 minutes.

6 Arrange the baked tofu and vegetables on a plate and garnish with bean sprouts, cilantro leaves, red chili, and a good squeeze of lime juice.

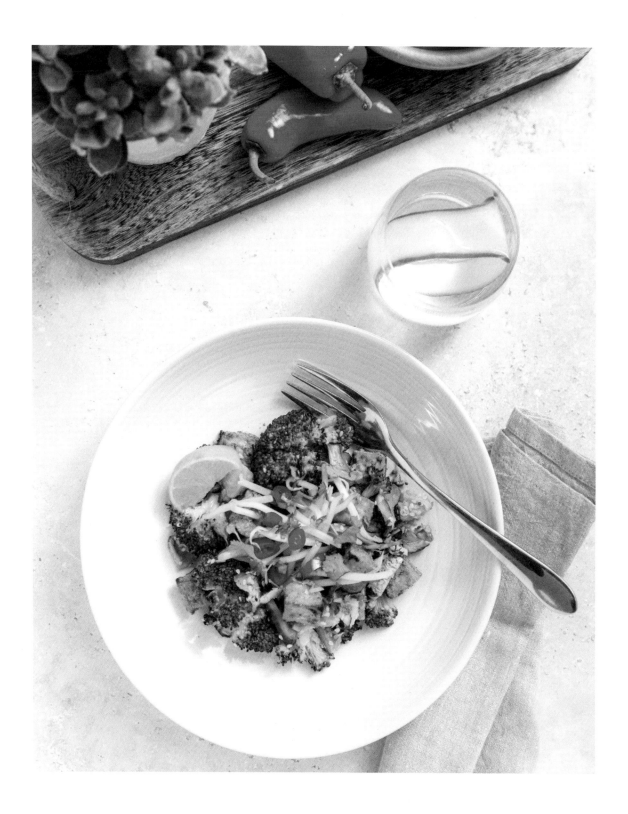

CHICKEN KATSU

SERVES ONE

1 chicken breast, the size and thickness of your palm

1¾oz (50g) bulgur wheat (5½oz/150g cooked weight)

sprig of fresh cilantro, to garnish

FOR THE KATSU SAUCE

1 tsp coconut oil

¼ cup minced red onion

1 garlic clove, finely chopped

½ tsp grated fresh ginger root

½ tsp garam masala

½ tsp mild curry powder

1 heaping tsp full-fat Greek yogurt OR Greek-style soy-based vegan yogurt

squeeze of lemon juice

It is the katsu sauce that makes this dish—the coconut and spices make it really feel like a treat, yet it's so simple to make and perfect for a Friday night at home! I also firmly believe that if your food looks good, it tastes good. For example, the bulgur wheat looks fabulous when you turn it out of a small cup into a dome shape. It's so easy to achieve, so try it!

1 Preheat the oven to 350°F.

2 Place the chicken in a medium-size ovenproof dish and bake in the oven for approximately 20 minutes until cooked through (see Good to Know).

3 While the chicken is cooking, prepare the bulgur wheat. Bring a small pan of water to a boil and cook it according to the package instructions (approximately 20 minutes), then drain and set aside.

4 Now, make the katsu sauce. Heat the coconut oil in a non-stick saute pan over low heat and gently saute the onion, garlic, and ginger for 5 minutes.

5 Add the garam masala and curry powder and stir, then add a generous ⅓ cup (100 ml) water and stir again. Bring to a boil, then reduce the heat and stir in the Greek yogurt and a squeeze of lemon juice. Take off the heat and blend to a smooth consistency.

6 Pack the bulgur wheat into the mold of a small cup, then turn it out onto a plate. With a sharp knife, slice the chicken breast diagonally, then arrange the pieces on the plate and spoon over the katsu sauce. Garnish with a sprig of cilantro and serve.

GOOD TO KNOW

You can bake or broil your chicken. Either way, it will take you around 20 minutes. Remember to turn your chicken over halfway through to allow the breast to cook evenly. If you want your chicken to remain juicy and make it easier to slice, cover with foil and rest for 5 minutes.

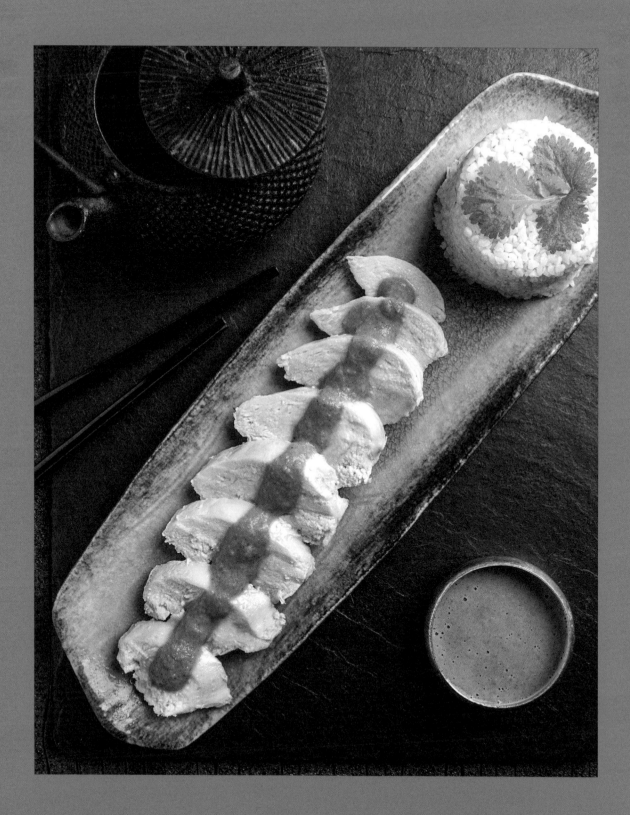

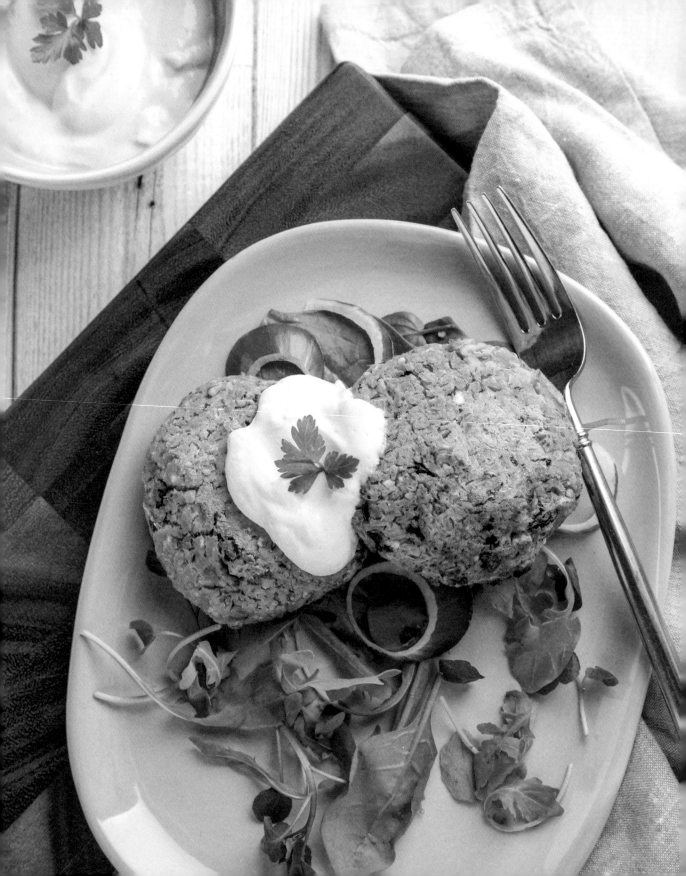

VEGAN FISH CAKES
WITH PLANT-BASED GARLIC MAYONNAISE

handful of chopped sweet potato

15oz (425g) can of butter beans, rinsed and drained

1 garlic clove, crushed

1 shallot

1 heaping tsp finely chopped flat-leaf parsley, plus an extra sprig to garnish

1 red chili (deseeded if you don't like too much heat)

½ tsp paprika

½ tsp Italian seasoning

½ sheet of nori

2 tsp extra virgin olive oil

pinch of white pepper

FOR THE MAYONNAISE

10oz (300g) soft silken tofu

1–2 garlic cloves, crushed

½ tsp mustard powder

squeeze of lemon juice

splash of unsweetened soy milk or pea milk

TO SERVE

handful of salad leaves

½ red onion

wedge of lemon

Who needs fish for a fish cake when edible seaweed can provide that authentic, salty taste of the sea? And you must complete it by serving it with the delicious plant-based garlic mayo.

1 Preheat the oven to 350°F and line a baking sheet with foil or parchment paper.

2 Bring a pot of water to a boil and cook the sweet potato for around 20 minutes or until soft. When cooked, mash thoroughly until smooth, then set aside to cool.

3 Now, make the plant-based mayonnaise. Simply place all the ingredients in a blender and puree until smooth. While the potato is cooling, you can also prepare the rest of the filling.

4 In a food processor, place the butter beans, garlic, shallot, parsley, chili, paprika, Italian seasoning, nori, olive oil, and white pepper and blend to a coarse mix. Add the cooled potato to the food processor and combine thoroughly, until ready to make into patties.

5 Now for the fun part. Divide the mixture into four portions and shape into equal-sized patties. Place the fish cakes on the prepared baking sheet and bake in the oven for approximately 20 minutes, turning halfway through.

6 Arrange two fish cakes on each plate on a bed of salad leaves and scatter the sliced onion and parsley over them. Serve with a slice of lemon and a tablespoon of delicious, homemade, plant-based garlic mayo.

GOOD TO KNOW

The garlic mayo can be stored in an airtight container and will keep in the fridge for a few days. Alternatively, you can freeze it in freezer bags, and it will keep for up to a month.

GRILLED TOFU POKE BOWL

1oz (30g) bulgur wheat (2¾oz/80g cooked weight)

small handful of edamame beans

4 baby corn, cut in half

1 radish, thinly sliced

piece of soft tofu, the size and thickness of your palm, thinly sliced

½ avocado, thinly sliced

FOR THE DRESSING

½ tsp wasabi paste

2 tbsp plain sugar-free yogurt OR soy-based vegan yogurt

juice of ½ lime

½ tsp sesame oil

This brightly colored bowl of goodness is packed full of antioxidants, and the wasabi dressing adds a lovely fresh flavor punch!

1 Bring a small pan of water to a boil and cook the bulgur wheat according to the package instructions—about 20 minutes. Drain and set aside.

2 Place the edamame beans in a small saucepan and cover with boiling water for 10 minutes, before draining and leaving to cool.

3 Now, make the dressing. In a bowl, add the wasabi paste, yogurt, lime juice, and sesame oil, and mix to combine.

4 Spoon the cooked bulgur wheat onto a plate and top with all the remaining ingredients. Drizzle the dressing over it, reserving extra for dunking. Serve with chopsticks!

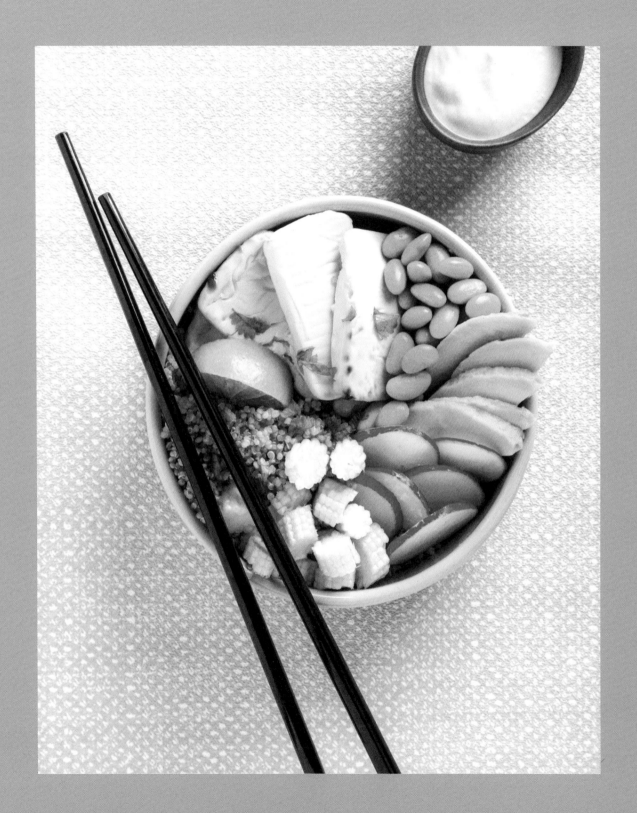

SALMON AND GOJI BERRY CURRY

SERVES TWO

2 salmon fillets (the size of your palm), skin removed and flesh cut into cubes

2½oz (75g) bulgur wheat (225g cooked weight)

2 tsp extra virgin olive oil

½ tsp cumin seeds

½ tsp mustard seeds

½ tsp coriander seeds

1 garlic clove

1 tsp grated fresh ginger root

½ tsp turmeric

2 tsp goji berries

1 tsp curry leaves

½ fresh chili, deseeded and finely chopped

3 tsp tomato paste

handful of arugula, to serve

1 tsp fresh, finely chopped cilantro, to garnish (optional)

wedge of lemon, to serve

The goji berry is such a great ingredient to include in your diet, as it provides so many benefits. It's good for the immune system, removes toxins from the body, promotes healthy skin, helps stabilize blood sugars, and can improve anxiety, depression, and sleep, to name a few. These little red berries have a sweet, slightly sour taste, which complements the salmon in this spicy tomato-based curry. This is seriously one of my best dishes!

1 First, remove the skin of your salmon and cut into cubes.

2 Bring a small pan of water to a boil and cook the bulgur wheat according to the package instructions—around 20 minutes. Drain and set aside.

3 Meanwhile, heat the olive oil in a non-stick saute pan over medium heat and fry the cumin, mustard, and coriander seeds until they become fragrant and start to pop. Remove from the heat and transfer to a bowl to allow to cool a little.

4 Return the pan to the stovetop and gently saute the garlic with the ginger and turmeric for 2 minutes, stirring all the time to ensure everything gets a nice coating in the flavored oil.

5 Add the goji berries, curry leaves, chili, and tomato paste to the spices, along with a generous ⅓ cup (100ml) water. Bring to a boil, stirring, then reduce the heat and simmer for 3 minutes.

6 Fold the salmon cubes gently into the sauce and simmer for an additional 5 minutes.

7 Spoon the bulgur wheat onto a plate with a small handful of arugula and spoon the curry on top. Finish with a garnish of cilantro (if using) and serve with a wedge of lemon.

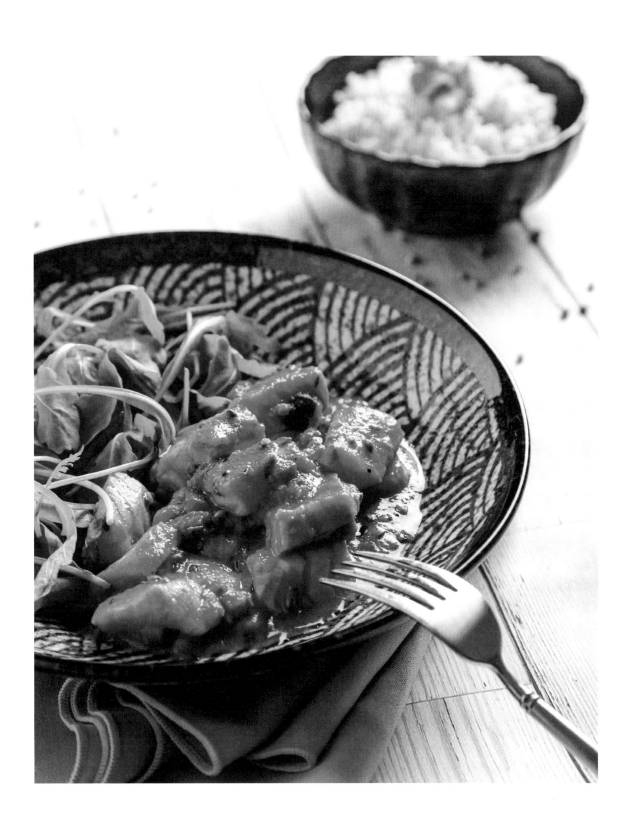

STUFFED ROASTED PEPPERS

 SERVES ONE

1 red or yellow pepper

1 tsp extra virgin olive oil

½ red onion, finely chopped

1 garlic clove, finely chopped

1 tsp ground ginger

pinch of cumin seeds

1 tsp ground coriander

1 tsp tomato paste

15oz (425g) can of chickpeas, drained and rinsed

handful of fresh, finely chopped cilantro, plus an extra sprig to garnish

2 tsp golden raisins

zest of 1 lime

Peppers are full of vitamins C, E, and beta-carotene, and roasting them creates such an incredible flavor. If you then stuff them, you can add even more flavor and extra nutrition.

1 Preheat the oven to 400°F.

2 Prepare the bell pepper by slicing off the top (reserving it for later) and removing the seeds inside. Place the pepper on a baking sheet and roast in the oven for 20 minutes.

3 Finely chop the top of the pepper and place in a non-stick saute pan with the olive oil, onion, and garlic. Cook, stirring, until soft and caramelized, then stir in the spices and cook until fragrant.

4 Add the tomato paste, chickpeas, cilantro, and golden raisins with a generous ⅓ cup (100ml) water. Bring to a boil, then reduce to a simmer and cook for another 5 minutes.

5 Place the roasted pepper on a plate and fill with the spiced chickpea mixture. Garnish with a scattering of chopped cilantro and lime zest, and enjoy!

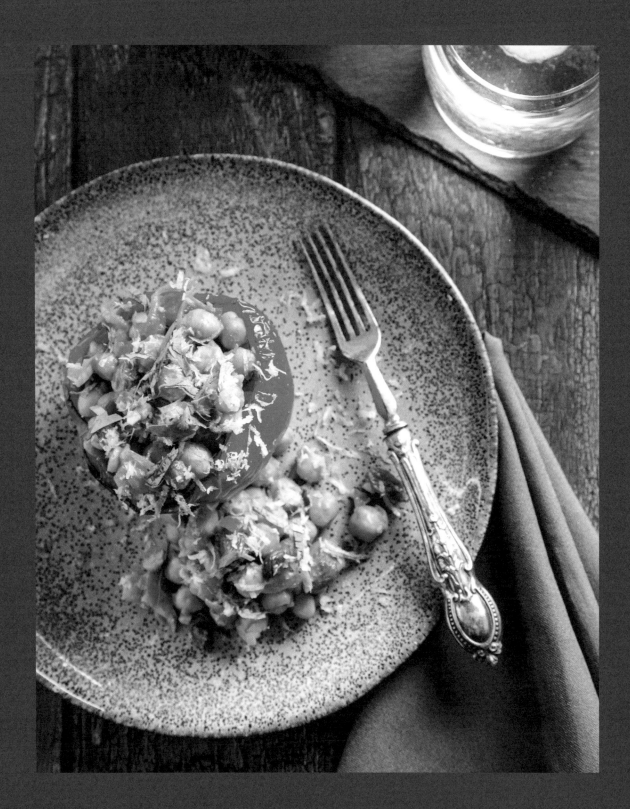

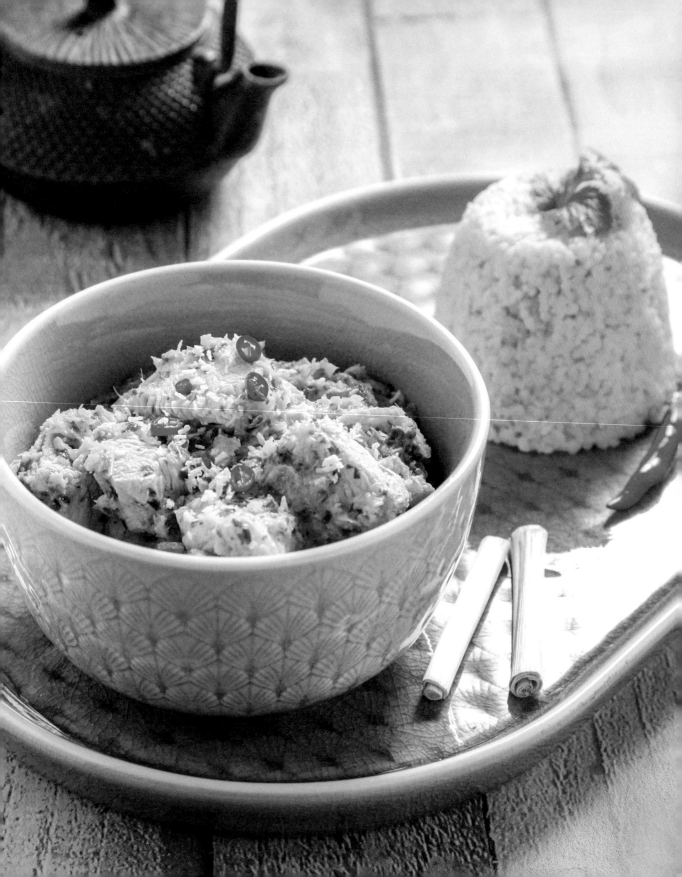

THAI GREEN CURRY

SERVES TWO

1 tsp coconut oil

4 tbsp coconut milk

2 chicken breast fillets, the size and thickness of your palm, cubed

2½oz (75g) dry bulgur wheat (225g cooked weight)

pinch of white pepper

juice of ½ lemon

juice of ½ lime

pinch of dried, shredded coconut, to garnish

FOR THE CURRY PASTE

handful of fresh cilantro, plus extra to garnish

2 sticks of lemongrass, chopped

1 thumb-size piece of fresh ginger, grated

2 fresh makrut lime leaves (or dry, if you can't find fresh)

1 Thai red chili, finely chopped, plus extra to garnish

½ small red onion, chopped

1 garlic clove, crushed

zest of ½ lime

1 tsp extra virgin olive oil

I love Thai food, and this curry is one of my most popular recipes. The bold flavors of lemongrass, garlic, and ginger never fail to satisfy, plus they're rich in beneficial nutrients. Coconut milk brings the whole curry together and makes it truly indulgent, as good as what you'd get in a restaurant!

1   Ideally, make the curry paste in a small food processor (or with a pestle and mortar). Place all the ingredients together and puree into a rough paste.

2   Heat the coconut oil in a non-stick pan over medium heat and cook the curry paste, stirring to release all the flavors.

3   Add a splash of water, stir, and then add the coconut milk and mix until combined.

4   Add the chicken, bring to a boil, and simmer for 10 minutes.

5   While the curry is simmering, prepare the bulgur wheat according to the package instructions.

6   Add the white pepper, lemon, and lime juice and stir the curry sauce. Cook for another 5 minutes, or until the chicken is cooked through.

7   Portion the curry and bulgur wheat beautifully on a plate and garnish with the remaining fresh coriander, chili, and a scattering of dried, shredded coconut.

MENEMEN

SERVES TWO

2 tsp extra virgin olive oil

1 onion, finely chopped

1 green pepper, finely chopped

½ tsp paprika

½ tsp cayenne pepper

1 tsp dried oregano

14oz (411g) can of chopped tomatoes

1 tsp capers, roughly chopped

freshly ground black pepper

piece of firm tofu, 3 x the size and thickness of your palm, crumbled

FOR THE DRESSING

2 tbsp plain sugar-free yogurt OR soy-based vegan yogurt

¼ tsp finely chopped garlic

½ tsp finely chopped chives

This traditional Turkish dish is basically scrambled eggs with tomatoes, peppers, and onion, flavored with delicious spices and drizzled with yogurt. Here, I've replaced the eggs with scrambled tofu to create a very similar effect, but you can use eggs, if you prefer. This dish is punchy with flavor and super-speedy, and it makes a great meal for any time of the day.

1 Heat the olive oil in a non-stick saute pan and saute the onion and pepper with the paprika, cayenne pepper, and oregano. Add a splash of water and cook for around 8 minutes, until the vegetables are soft.

2 Add the tomatoes and capers with a good grind of black pepper, then stir in the crumbled tofu and cook for another 4 minutes.

3 Now, make the dressing. Place the yogurt, garlic, and chives in a small bowl and mix well.

4 Divide the menemen between two bowls and serve with a tablespoon of the delicious garlic dressing on top.

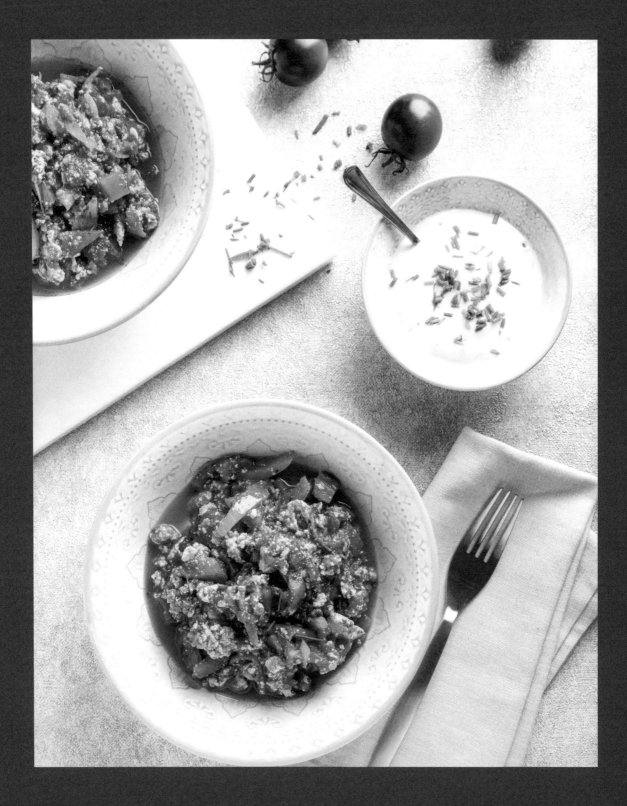

SASHIMI BOWL

1 sushi-grade, palm-sized tuna fillet, thinly sliced

handful of cooked green beans, chopped

handful of shredded red cabbage

handful of thinly sliced radish

handful of edamame beans

handful of thinly sliced red pepper

handful of grated raw beetroot

1 green onion, finely sliced, to garnish

sesame seeds, to garnish

FOR THE DRESSING

1 tsp sesame oil

juice of $\frac{1}{4}$ lime

$\frac{1}{2}$ garlic clove, crushed

$\frac{1}{4}$ tsp grated fresh ginger root

1 tsp coconut milk

$\frac{1}{4}$ fresh chili, finely chopped (optional)

If you love the delicate flavors of Japanese food, then you will love this fresh, vibrant, and beautifully presented dish of tuna and vegetables, all ready to be dipped in the zesty dressing. Edamame are quite simply soybeans, and they are a great ingredient—full of fiber and protein.

1 This dish is all about the presentation. Take your favorite bowl and, working in a circular motion, spread out the ingredients one by one, starting with the tuna. Scatter the green onion and sesame seeds over everything.

2 Now, make the dressing. In a bowl, place all the ingredients and stir to combine. You can either drizzle this over the sashimi bowl or use it as a dip.

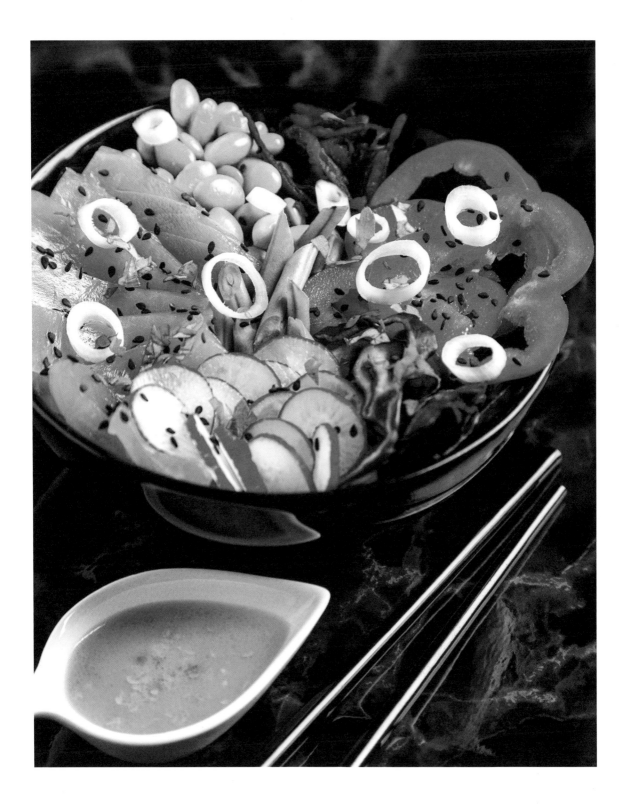

QUESADILLAS

SERVES ONE

handful of diced sweet potato

15oz (425g) can of black beans, drained and rinsed

1 tsp smoked paprika

1 tsp Cajun spice

handful of fresh, finely chopped cilantro, plus extra to garnish

juice and zest of 1 lime, plus an extra wedge to garnish

1 whole-wheat tortilla

FOR THE SMASHED AVOCADO

½ avocado

1 red pepper, finely chopped

juice and zest of ½ lime

pinch of chili flakes

FOR THE SALSA

1 tsp extra virgin olive oil

2 garlic cloves

handful of fresh, finely chopped basil

1 tbsp tomato paste

14oz (411g) can of chopped tomatoes

freshly ground black pepper

No cheese? No problem! My vegan quesadillas are rich with black beans, smooth with smashed avocado, and zingy with tomato salsa... Olé!

1 Bring a pan of water to a boil and cook the sweet potato for around 10 minutes, until soft, then drain and set aside in a large bowl.

2 In a large bowl, place the black beans, paprika, Cajun spice, cilantro, and lime zest and juice, and mix together roughly with a fork—you want a little texture, not a smooth paste. Spread the mixture across the whole-wheat tortilla and fold to make a sandwich.

3 Now, make the smashed avocado. Place all the ingredients in a bowl and mash with a fork to combine.

4 Now, make the salsa. Heat the olive oil in a saute pan and saute the garlic over low heat. Add the basil and tomato paste and cook, stirring, for 2 minutes, then add the canned tomatoes, season with black pepper, and simmer for 10–15 minutes to let the flavors combine and the tomatoes break down.

5 In a dry, non-stick pan over medium heat, cook the quesadilla for 2 minutes on each side, until crisp and golden. Serve with your smashed avocado, tomato salsa, and a wedge of lime and garnish with a sprig of cilantro.

GOOD TO KNOW

The tomato salsa can be stored in an airtight container and will keep in the fridge for a few days. Alternatively, you can freeze it in freezer bags, and it will keep for up to a month.

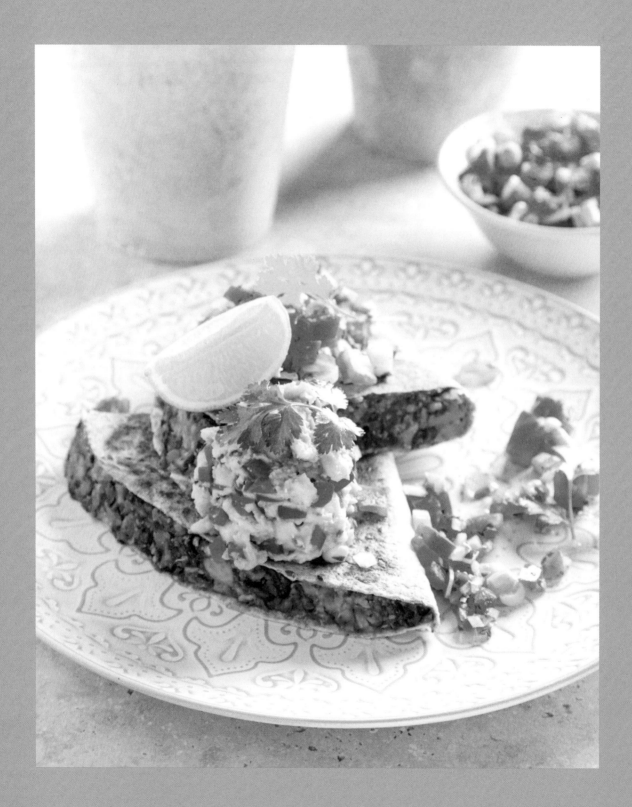

ASIAN PILAF / SERVES TWO

2 tsp extra virgin olive oil

½ tsp cumin seeds

3 cardamom pods

1 cinnamon stick

1 tsp grated fresh ginger

½ red chili, finely chopped

1 garlic clove, finely chopped

½ red onion, finely chopped

½ tsp ground turmeric

1 tsp garam masala

large handful of mixed vegetables (can be frozen)

piece of firm tofu, 3 x the size and thickness of your palm

1⅓oz (40g) bulgur wheat (3½oz/100g cooked weight)

pinch of white pepper

1 heaping tbsp fresh, finely chopped cilantro, plus a little extra to garnish

juice of ½ lemon

1 tbsp pomegranate seeds

2 lemon wedges, to serve

A pilaf is a one-pot rice dish from the Middle East and Asia that's bursting with flavor! I love its versatility, as it provides the basis for so many flavor variations. Here, I'm using heart-healthy bulgur wheat, as it's full of fiber and nutrients. Add the pomegranate seeds for extra antioxidants and a sweet-sour crunch.

1 Heat the olive oil in a large non-stick saute pan over medium-high heat and cook the cumin, cardamom, and cinnamon until beautifully fragrant.

2 Turn the heat down to low and add the ginger, chili, and garlic, along with a splash of water to bring all the flavors together. Warm through for a minute.

3 Add the onion and cook to soften, then stir in the turmeric and garam masala.

4 Add the vegetables and tofu and stir until nicely coated, then cook for 5–8 minutes. If necessary, add another splash of water to keep the spices from sticking to the bottom of the pan.

5 Keeping the pan over low heat, add the bulgur wheat and stir to combine. Pour in 1¼ cups (300ml) water with a pinch of pepper and half the chopped cilantro and stir again. Bring the pan to a boil, then reduce to a simmer and cook for 10 minutes, until the bulgur wheat has absorbed the liquid but still retains a slight bite (you don't want it too soft).

6 Take the pan off the heat and stir in the lemon juice and pomegranate seeds. Remove the cinnamon stick and cardamom pods and then divide between two plates and garnish with a little cilantro and a wedge of lemon.

CHICKEN KEBAB
WITH **BABA GHANOUSH**

SERVES ONE

1 chicken breast, the size and
thickness of your palm, cut
into cubes

½ large red pepper, cut into
large pieces

½ large red onion, cut into
large pieces

freshly ground black pepper

squeeze of lemon juice

small handful of arugula or
mixed salad leaves

FOR THE MARINADE

1 tsp extra virgin olive oil

1 garlic clove, finely chopped

1 heaping tsp full-fat Greek
yogurt OR Greek-style soy-based
vegan yogurt

¼ tsp paprika

½ tsp Italian seasoning

FOR THE BABA GHANOUSH

1 small purple eggplant

juice of ½ lemon

1 small garlic clove

pinch of onion powder

pinch of ground cumin

pinch of finely chopped
flat-leaf parsley

My chicken kebab uses a simple, flavorsome marinade to elevate your average chicken dish. When you serve it with a delicious homemade baba ghanoush, you get to taste a little bit of Lebanese heaven!

1 First, make the marinade. Place all the ingredients in a large bowl and mix together. Add the chicken, red pepper, and onion pieces and turn to coat thoroughly. Cover the bowl and refrigerate overnight, if possible, to really let the marinade soak in, or for at least 2 hours. However, if you just can't wait, then go for it.

2 When you are ready to cook, preheat one oven to 350°F and preheat the broiler on a second oven, with the rack placed halfway up. You can also use a BBQ grill.

3 Make the baba ghanoush. With a fork, prick the eggplant all over to ensure steam can escape when cooking, then place on a wire rack and cook in the preheated oven for 30 minutes. When cool enough to handle, scoop out the soft flesh and transfer to a blender with all the remaining ingredients. Blend until you have the consistency you like.

4 Meanwhile, thread the marinated chicken, red pepper, and red onion onto a long skewer and season with black pepper and a squeeze of lemon. Arrange the kebabs on a baking sheet and place under the broiler for approximately 15–20 minutes, turning frequently, until cooked through. If using a BBQ grill, place on the grill and cook for 10–15 minutes, turning once.

5 Serve the kebab with fresh arugula or salad leaves and an additional squeeze of lemon juice, accompanied by a spoonful of baba ghanoush.

GOOD TO KNOW

The baba ghanoush can be stored in an airtight container and will keep in the fridge for a few days. Alternatively, you can freeze it in freezer bags, and it will keep for up to a month.

TANDOORI SALMON KEBABS

SERVES TWO

1 heaping tsp full-fat Greek yogurt OR Greek-style soy-based vegan yogurt

½ tsp ground cumin

½ tsp ground coriander

¼ tsp ground ginger

1 tsp garam masala

½ tsp mild chili powder

¼ tsp white pepper

2 tsp extra virgin olive oil

2 salmon fillets (the size and thickness of your palm)

½ red onion, roughly chopped

2 whole-wheat tortillas

4 Little Gem lettuce leaves, shredded

4 cherry tomatoes, quartered

handful of fresh, finely chopped cilantro, to garnish

wedge of lemon, to serve

FOR THE SPICY MINT SAUCE

handful of fresh, finely chopped cilantro

handful of fresh, finely chopped mint

zest and juice of ½ lemon

½ tsp cumin seeds

1 green chili, deseeded and finely chopped

1 garlic clove, crushed

2 green onions, chopped

3 tbsp full-fat Greek yogurt OR Greek-style soy-based vegan yogurt

The inspiration for this salmon dish is straightforward. Strong aromatic tandoori spices combined with a cool but spicy mint sauce makes for a flavor explosion—it's so good!

1 First, make the tandoori paste for the marinade. In a wide bowl, place the yogurt, spices, and oil and mix to combine. Add the salmon fillets and onion to the bowl and turn in the marinade until thoroughly coated. Place in the fridge to marinate, ideally overnight.

2 Preheat the oven to 350°F.

3 Now, make the spicy mint sauce. Place all the ingredients in a blender and puree to a smooth paste.

4 Place the marinated salmon on a baking sheet and bake in the oven for approximately 15 minutes or until cooked, turning halfway through.

5 Place a tortilla wrap on two serving plates and divide the lettuce and tomatoes between them. When the salmon is cooked, lay a fillet on top of each wrap and drizzle all over with the spicy mint sauce. Garnish with cilantro and serve with a wedge of lemon for squeezing. The salmon can be wrapped in the tortilla if you like— your choice!

GOOD TO KNOW

The mint sauce can be stored in an airtight container and will keep in the fridge for a few days. Alternatively, you can freeze it in freezer bags, and it will keep for up to a month.

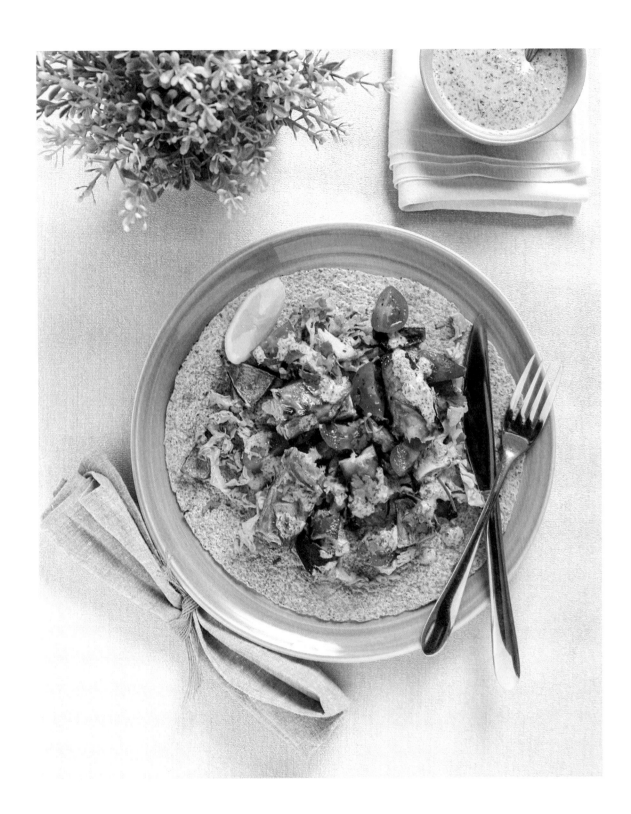

SWEET POTATO JACKET WITH CORONATION CHICKEN

1 sweet potato, the size of your hand

1 chicken breast fillet, the size and thickness of your palm

finely chopped cilantro, to garnish

FOR THE CORONATION SAUCE

½ tbsp full-fat Greek yogurt

½ tsp curry powder

¼ tsp ground cinnamon

pinch of white pepper

2 tsp flaked almonds, crushed

2 tsp golden raisins

Feast like royalty! This Coronation chicken recipe is a breeze to make and is the perfect topping for your baked sweet potato—a tasty, quick, and easy midweek dinner!

1 Preheat the oven to 400°F.

2 Place the sweet potato on an oven tray and bake in the oven for 40 minutes or until crispy on the outside and soft in the middle.

3 Meanwhile, poach the chicken for the filling. Place the chicken breast in a non-stick saucepan and cover with plenty of water. Bring to a boil, then reduce the heat to a simmer, and poach for 15–20 minutes, until the chicken is cooked through.

4 Now, make the creamy Coronation sauce. In a bowl, place the yogurt, curry powder, cinnamon, white pepper, almonds, and golden raisins and mix together thoroughly. Slice the chicken into bite-size pieces and turn in the sauce until coated.

5 Your potato should now be crispy on the outside and fluffy on the inside. Arrange on a plate, slice across the top lengthwise, and pinch until it opens to receive the delicious filling. Spoon the Coronation chicken on top and garnish with the cilantro.

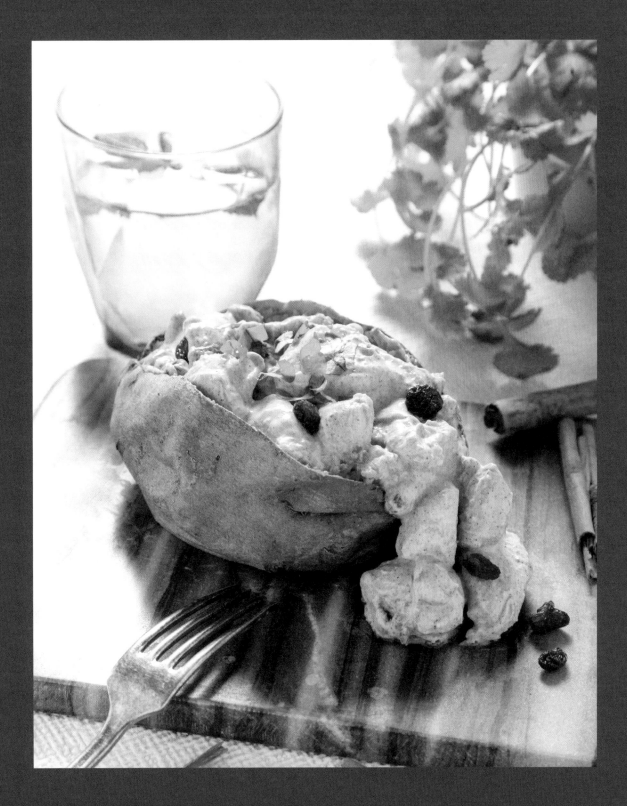

SUPER SALMON SALAD

SERVES TWO

2 salmon fillets, the size and thickness of your palm

1¾oz (50g) cracked freekeh (150g pre-cooked weight)

½ yellow (bell) pepper

½ small cucumber

8 cherry tomatoes, quartered

½ carrot, grated

1 avocado, chopped

freshly ground black pepper

squeeze of lemon

1 tbsp fresh, finely chopped cilantro

Freekeh is a type of nutrient-rich whole grain that is made from young wheat and is integral to Middle Eastern and North African cuisine. It is similar to bulgur wheat or quinoa, which you could also use here, and has a lovely chewy, nutty texture and smoky flavor. Freekeh that is cracked is easier to cook, but you could use any type—pre-cooked is the easiest of all!

1 Preheat the oven to 400°F and line a baking sheet with parchment paper.

2 Place the salmon on the prepared tray and cook for 15–20 minutes, according to your preferences. Meanwhile, bring a pot of water to a boil and cook the freekeh according to the package instructions, about 20 minutes.

3 Place the pepper, cucumber, tomatoes, carrot, and avocado in a bowl. When the freekeh is cooked, fluff it up with a fork and then add to the salad ingredients. Flake the cooked salmon into the bowl and toss everything together.

4 Season with black pepper and a squeeze of lemon, toss again, and then garnish with fresh cilantro.

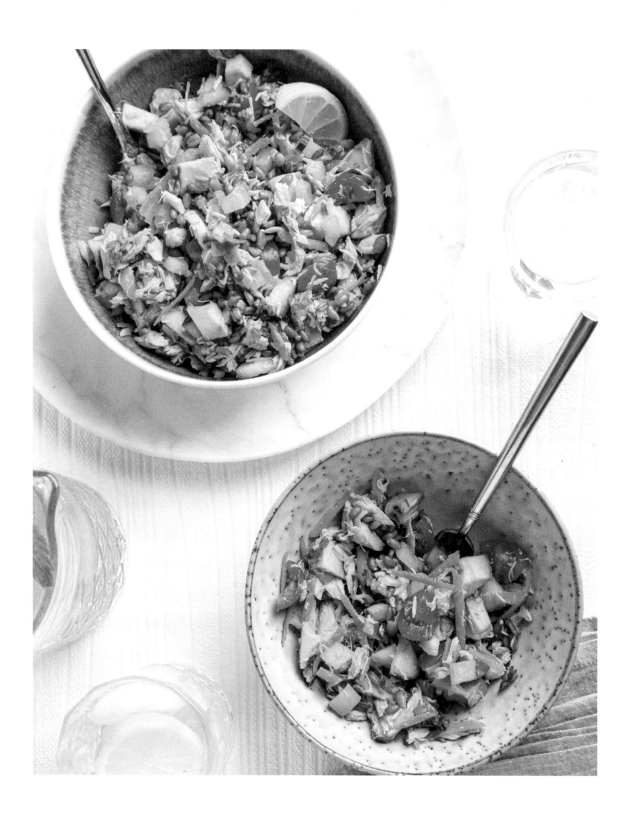

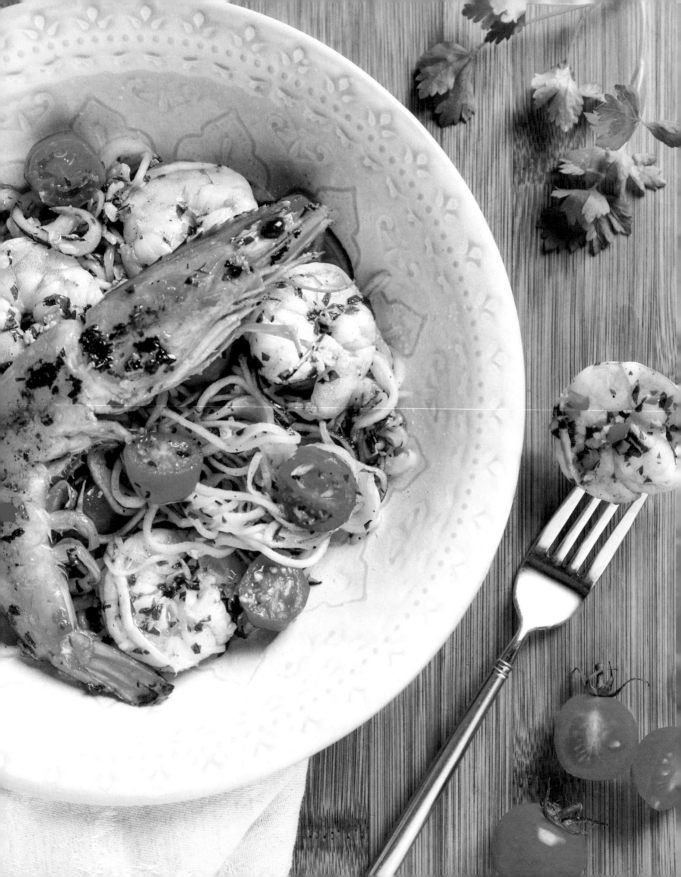

GARLIC AND CHILI LARGE SHRIMP SINGUINE

SERVES TWO

1 zucchini
zest of 1 lemon
freshly ground black pepper
2 tsp extra virgin olive oil
½ chili, deseeded and finely chopped
3 garlic cloves, crushed
1 tbsp finely chopped flat-leaf parsley, plus extra to garnish
2 large handfuls of raw large shrimp (2 x the size and thickness of your palm)
4 cherry tomatoes, cut in half
juice of ½ lemon

There's a reason this delicious Mediterranean pasta dish is a classic, and also one of my favorite dishes to make. Parsley is known as the balancing herb, and it brightens the flavor of the shrimp, while slightly toning down the strong impact of the garlic and chili. Substituting zucchini noodles for traditional pasta is also a great way to add even more nutrients.

1 Using a spiralizer, turn your zucchini into zucchini noodles. Alternatively, you can julienne the zucchini into thin strips or use a vegetable peeler to create long ribbons, like tagliatelle.

2 Place the zucchini noodles into a bowl and toss with lemon zest and black pepper, then set aside.

3 Heat the olive oil in a non-stick saute pan over low heat and cook the chili, garlic, and parsley for a couple of minutes, until aromatic. Add the shrimp and tomatoes and cook, stirring, for 5 minutes or until the shrimp turns pink. Turn off the heat.

4 Add the lemon juice and stir, then drop in the zucchini noodles and toss everything in the pan together to combine. Serve in a large pasta bowl and garnish with a little extra chopped parsley.

GOOD TO KNOW

I like to use frozen raw shrimp, which I defrost overnight in my fridge – they taste just as good as fresh shrimp, and they're often cheaper. Also, don't forget to de-vein your shrimp – simply make a small slice down the middle of the back with a sharp knife to expose the dark vein and remove.

MEXICAN BLACK BEAN CHILI

SERVES TWO

2 tsp extra virgin olive oil

1 small onion, finely chopped

1 red pepper, finely chopped

2 garlic cloves, finely chopped

½ red chili, finely chopped

1 tsp ground cumin

1 tsp ground coriander

1 tsp paprika

3 tbsp tomato paste

½ cup (90g) dried red split lentils

15oz (425g) can of black beans, drained and rinsed

fresh, finely chopped cilantro, to garnish

A warming, homemade chili is one of my favorite types of comfort food, and this plant-based version is so full of nutrition and flavor and easy to whip up—in less than 30 minutes.

1 Heat the olive oil in a large non-stick saute pan over low to medium heat and cook the onion and pepper until softened. Add the garlic, chili, and spices and stir everything together until combined.

2 Add the tomato paste with 1¾ cups (400ml) water, then bring to a boil. Reduce the heat, add the lentils, and simmer in the juices for around 10 minutes, until softened. Finally, add the black beans and cook until warmed through.

3 Garnish with chopped cilantro and serve.

CHICKEN MADRAS
WITH **QUINOA**

SERVES ONE

1 tsp coconut oil

½ red onion, finely chopped

½ red pepper, finely chopped

1 garlic clove, finely chopped

1 tsp grated fresh ginger root

3 cloves

3 cardamom pods, cracked

1 chicken fillet, the size and thickness of your palm, cut into cubes

½ tsp turmeric

½ tsp ground cumin

½ tsp ground coriander

¼ tsp chili powder

pinch of white pepper

1 heaping tsp tomato paste

1oz (30g) quinoa (90g cooked weight)

juice of ½ lemon

small handful of fresh, finely chopped cilantro, to garnish

This recipe is probably the easiest curry to make (ever!) and is full of pantry staples, so it's perfect for that midweek meal when you have very little left in the fridge. I love to eat quinoa with curry instead of rice, as the slightly nutty flavor works so well with all the spices, and it adds texture!

1 Heat the coconut oil in a large non-stick saute pan over low to medium heat and gently saute the onion, pepper, garlic, and ginger with the cloves and cardamom pods. Cook, stirring, for about 5 minutes, until the vegetables are soft.

2 Add the chicken and stir for a few minutes. Add the turmeric, cumin, ground coriander, chili powder, white pepper, and tomato paste with 3½ tablespoons water and stir again to combine. Bring to a boil, then reduce the heat and simmer for 15 minutes or until the chicken is cooked through.

3 While the curry is simmering, prepare the quinoa according to the package instructions.

4 When the chicken is cooked, stir in the lemon juice. Spoon the quinoa onto a serving plate and top with the curry (you may want to remove the cardamom pods and cloves). Garnish with cilantro and serve.

DELICIOUS DHAL

SERVES THREE

10oz (300g) dry red lentils, rinsed

3 tsp extra virgin olive oil

1 red onion, finely chopped

2 garlic cloves, crushed

14oz (411g) can of chopped tomatoes

1 tbsp tomato paste

1 tsp turmeric

1 tsp cumin seeds

1 tsp ground coriander

1 tsp garam masala

1 tsp fresh ginger root

pinch of chili flakes

pinch of white pepper

3 whole-wheat wraps

handful of fresh, finely chopped cilantro, to garnish

wedge of lime, to serve

I love dhal—it's a plant-based, gluten-free, one-pot wonder and so easy to make. Even if you are not a fan of too much spice, the addition of tomatoes completely balances the flavors.

1 Place the rinsed lentils in a pot and cover with double the quantity of water. Bring to a boil, then reduce the heat and simmer for about 10 minutes, until soft. Drain and set aside.

2 Meanwhile, heat the oil in a large non-stick saute pan over medium heat and saute the onion and garlic until soft.

3 Add the tomatoes, tomato paste, spices, fresh ginger, chili flakes, and white pepper, along with the lentils, and simmer for 10 minutes while continuing to stir regularly.

4 Place another saute pan over medium heat and fry the whole-wheat wraps until crispy. You will have to watch them, as they can burn quickly. Cook one at a time, then cut into quarters and cover to keep warm.

5 Serve garnished with fresh cilantro and a wedge of lime, and use the crispy wraps in place of cutlery.

GOOD TO KNOW

You can microwave your whole-wheat wraps. Just place in the microwave for 20–30 seconds – they will be warm but not crispy.

Dhal also freezes very well so simply double the quantities if you want to make a big batch.

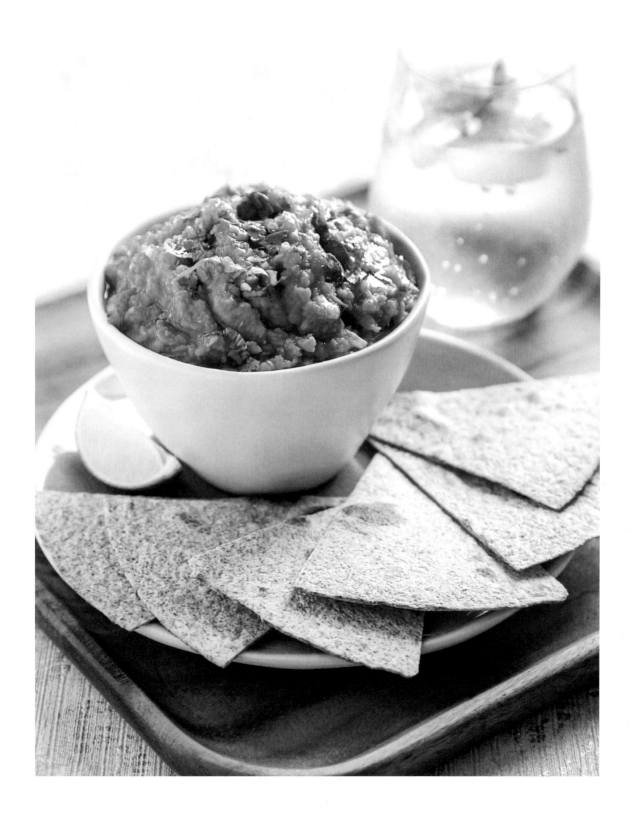

BLACK BEAN BAD BOY

SERVES TWO

¹/₄ cup (50g) bulgur wheat

1 tsp extra virgin olive oil

½ red onion, finely chopped

1 garlic clove, finely chopped

1 tsp ground cumin

15oz (425g) can of black beans, drained and rinsed

juice and zest of ½ lime

½ tsp paprika

piece of tofu, 1½ x the size and thickness of your palm, sliced

½ small ripe avocado, chopped

8 cherry tomatoes, quartered

½ red chili, thinly sliced, to garnish

handful of fresh, finely chopped cilantro, to garnish

wedge of lime, to serve

Black beans provide wonderful flavor and a full-on nutritional punch. I also love to cook with tofu—it's an excellent plant-based source of protein, rich in calcium and vitamin D, and naturally low in calories. It also has a very mild flavor, so it takes on whatever flavor it's paired with. I can't wait for you to try this bad boy!

1 First, prepare the bulgur wheat. Bring a pot of water to a boil and cook according to the package instructions—around 20 minutes—then drain and set aside.

2 Heat the olive oil in a saute pan over medium heat and saute the onion until soft. Turn down the heat and gently saute the garlic, stirring to ensure it doesn't burn. Stir in the cumin and cook until fragrant, then add the black beans and cook for 5 minutes. Stir in the lime zest and juice.

3 Now, preheat the broiler and prepare the tofu. Sprinkle the paprika over the tofu slices (this is important for adding flavor), then place under the broiler for 3–4 minutes on each side.

4 Place the bulgur wheat in a favorite bowl and top with the delicious black beans. Scatter the chopped avocado, tomatoes, and tofu over the top. Garnish with sliced chili and cilantro and serve with a wedge of lime.

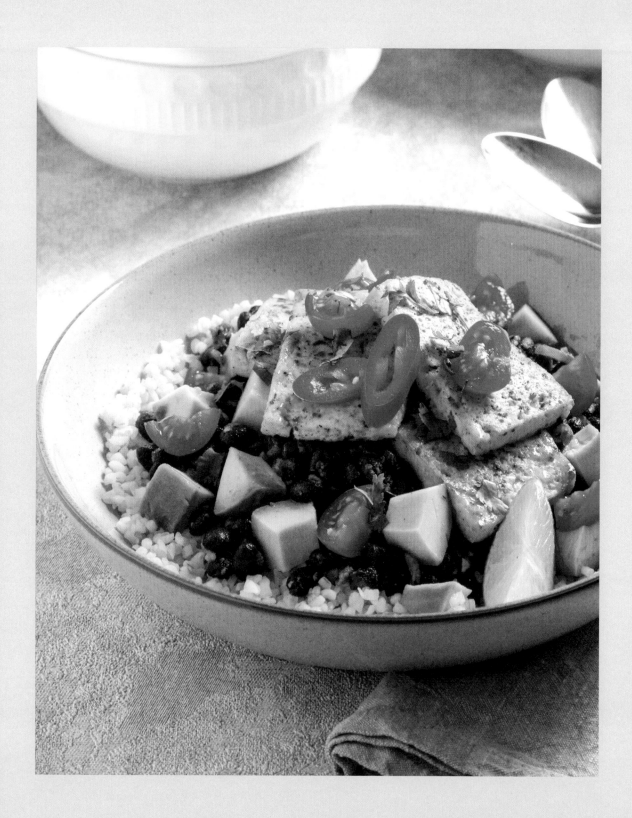

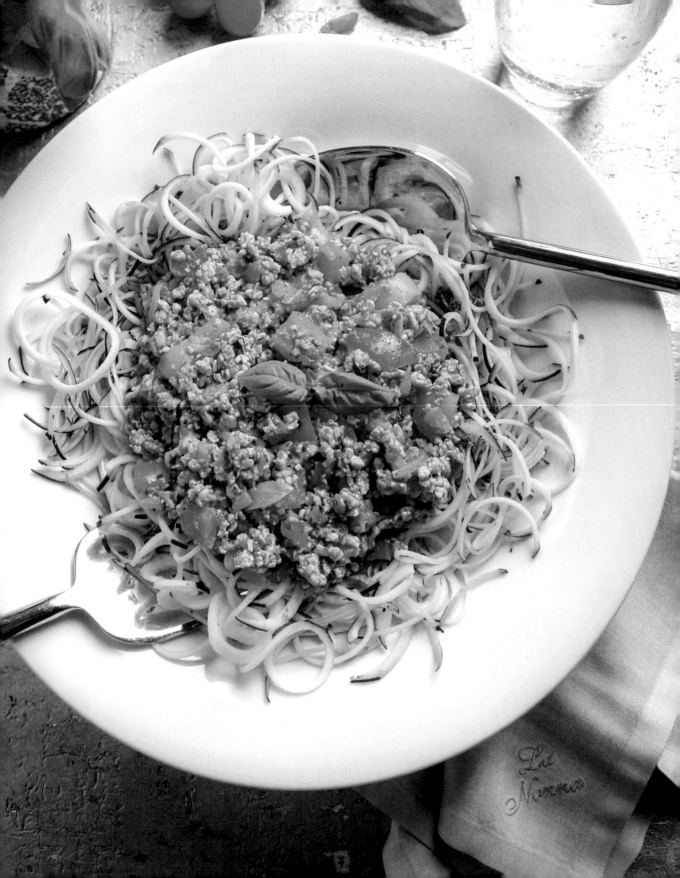

TURKEY BOLOGNESE

1 tsp extra virgin olive oil

1 red or yellow pepper, finely chopped

1 small red onion, finely chopped

2 garlic cloves, finely chopped

lean ground turkey, 2 x the size and thickness of your palm

6 olives, finely chopped

½ tsp white pepper

1 tsp mixed Italian herbs

12 fresh basil leaves, chopped, plus a sprig to garnish

1 tbsp tomato paste

14oz (411g) can of chopped tomatoes

1 zucchini, spiralized

This is how you make a traditional spaghetti Bolognese healthier—cook with a leaner protein (turkey) and swap out the carb-heavy pasta for nutrient-rich zucchini noodles.

1 Heat the olive oil in a large non-stick saute pan over medium heat and saute the pepper and onion until softened. Turn down the heat and gently saute the garlic, stirring to ensure it doesn't burn.

2 Add the ground turkey, olives, white pepper, Italian herbs, basil leaves, and tomato paste and cook until the turkey has browned.

3 Add the tomatoes, stir to combine and bring to a boil, then reduce the heat and simmer for 20 minutes.

4 In a non-stick skillet over low heat, saute the spiralized zucchini noodles for around 1–2 minutes or until they soften.

5 Heap a pile of zucchini noodles in a pasta bowl, spoon the turkey Bolognese on top, and garnish with a sprig of fresh basil.

CLASSIC BURGER

1 tsp flaxseed oil

½ white onion, finely chopped

1 garlic clove, finely chopped

½ tsp dried rosemary

½ tsp dried thyme

ground plant-based meat alternative, 1½ x the size and thickness of your palm

pinch of black pepper

4 cherry tomatoes

3 Little Gem lettuce leaves

½ red onion

FOR THE TOMATO KETCHUP

1 tbsp tomato paste

2 large pinches of white pepper

¼ tsp paprika

juice of ¼ lemon

freshly ground black pepper

We all love a burger, right? So, I had to create my super-healthy plant-based version that still has a satisfying bite! And swapping out the bun for a whole-wheat pita means that all the flavor of the patty takes center stage, and it's far easier to eat without all the toppings falling out—genius!

1 Preheat the oven to 350°F.

2 Heat the oil in a non-stick skillet over low to medium heat and cook the onion, garlic, rosemary, and thyme until soft.

3 Transfer the onion to a bowl and mix with the ground plant-based meat alternative until thoroughly combined. Season with black pepper and, with your hands, mold the mixture into a patty shape.

4 Preheat a ridged grill pan over medium heat and cook the burger for about 2 minutes on each side, until the edges brown. Transfer the pan to the oven and cook for another 10 minutes to make sure it is cooked through.

5 While the burger is cooking, make the tomato ketchup. Place all the ingredients in a small bowl with 4 tablespoons of water and stir until thoroughly combined.

6 Transfer the burger to a plate and keep warm. Place the cherry tomatoes on the hot grill pan and put them in the oven to roast until they begin to burst. At the same time, warm the pita in the oven.

7 When ready to serve, slice open the warmed pita, add the lettuce leaves, sliced red onion, and the delicious burger, and top with those bursting cherry tomatoes.

GOOD TO KNOW

Please do go the extra mile and make your own tomato ketchup so that it's full of natural ingredients and flavors rather than sugar and preservatives. It can be stored in an airtight container and will keep in the fridge for a few days. Alternatively, you can freeze it in freezer bags, and it will keep for up to a month.

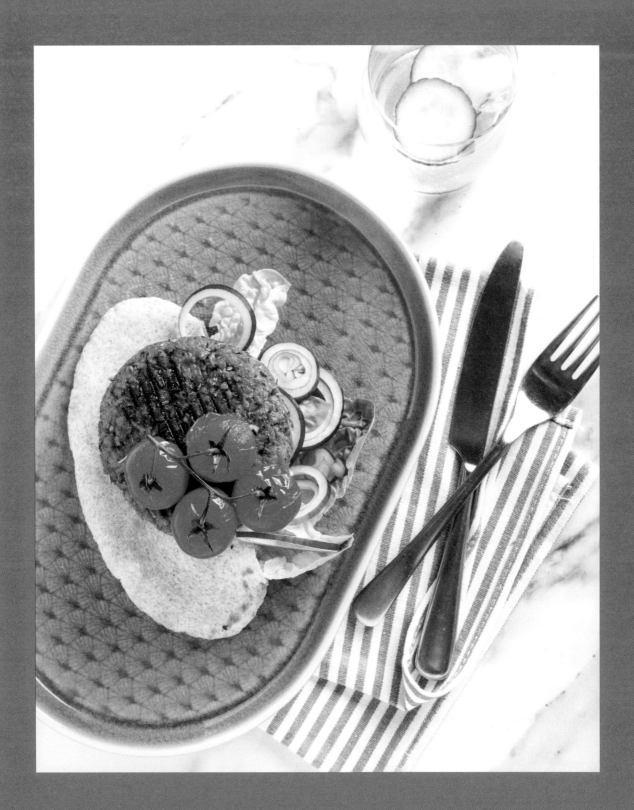

MOROCCAN CHICKEN TAGINE

1 tsp coconut oil

1 red pepper, chopped

½ small red onion, chopped

1 chicken breast, the size and thickness of your palm, cut into cubes

3 tsp ras el hanout

pinch of cinnamon

pinch of chili flakes

1 garlic clove, crushed

pinch of white pepper

1 tbsp tomato paste

1 tbsp fresh, finely chopped cilantro

handful of watercress or leafy salad

This tagine is so easy to make with just a handful of ingredients. The essential one here is ras el hanout, which is actually a mix of eight spices and provides the North African authenticity. I love to serve it with a handful of pungent, peppery watercress—an incredible superfood that contains significant amounts of iron as well as vitamins.

1 Heat the oil in a large non-stick saute pan over medium heat and saute the pepper and onion until soft. Add the chicken and cook, turning regularly until lightly browned all over.

2 Add the ras el hanout, cinnamon, chili flakes, garlic, and white pepper and stir the chicken until thoroughly coated in the aromatic spices. Add the tomato paste with a scant 2/3 cup (150ml) water and mix well to combine.

3 Simmer for 15–20 minutes, or until the chicken is cooked through. Serve garnished with some chopped cilantro and a handful of watercress or your favorite salad leaves.

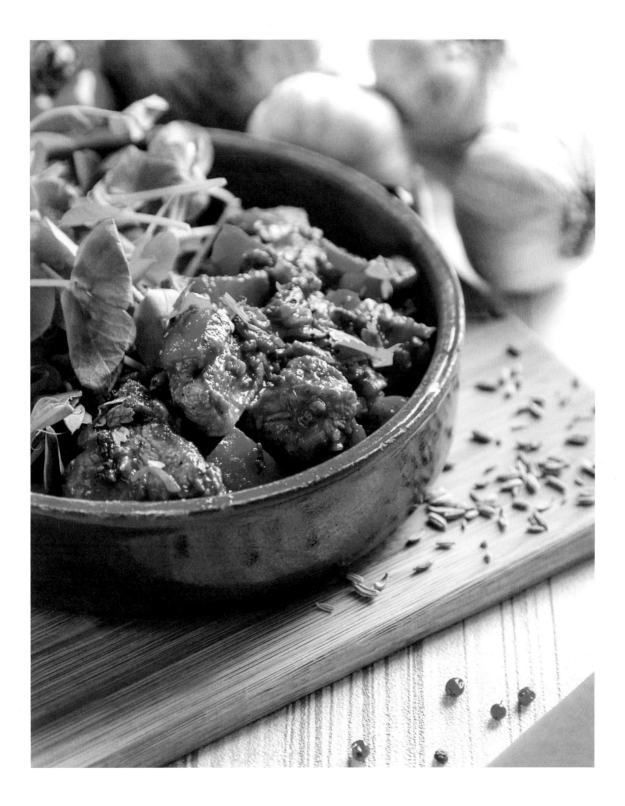

TUNA STEAK WITH A POMEGRANATE AND PAPAYA RELISH

SERVES TWO

2 tuna steaks, the size and thickness of your palm

1 tsp extra virgin olive oil

freshly ground black pepper

FOR THE RELISH

1 tsp extra virgin olive oil

½ cucumber, finely chopped

2 green onions, finely chopped

4 cherry tomatoes, quartered

½ red chili, deseeded and finely chopped

1 heaping tsp finely chopped flat-leaf parsley

1 heaping tbsp pomegranate seeds

1 heaping tbsp chopped papaya

juice of ½ lime

wedge of lime, to serve

A tuna steak is a little bit of a treat, so you want to cook it well (not too much!) and serve it with something delicious—like this beautifully colorful and fruity relish that tastes even better than it looks. I like mine just seared!

1 First, make the relish. Place all the ingredients in a bowl and stir to mix thoroughly.

2 Place a ridged grill pan over high heat to get hot. Brush both sides of each tuna steak with a little olive oil and season with black pepper. Place the fish on the griddle and cook for 1–2 minutes, then flip and cook for another 1–2 minutes on the other side. (I like my tuna rare. If you prefer yours more well done, cook for a little longer.)

3 Serve each tuna steak on a plate with spoonfuls of fruity relish and a wedge of lime to squeeze over it.

GOOD TO KNOW

You could also broil the tuna steaks under high heat, but I prefer a ridged grill pan, as it gives you those lines across the flesh, which makes for beautiful presentation!

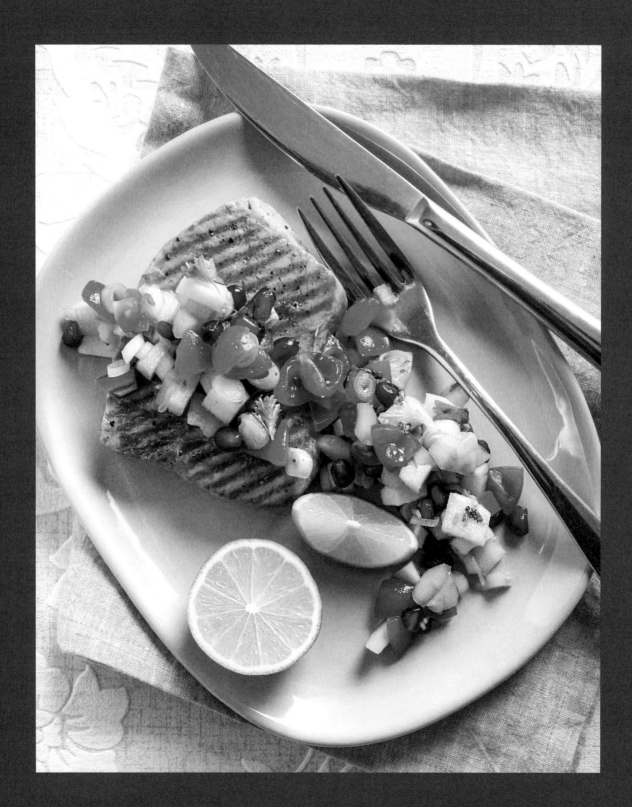

SESAME AND GINGER BOWL

zest and juice of 1 lime

1 tsp sesame seeds

1 thumb-size piece of fresh ginger, grated

1 garlic clove, finely chopped

handful of fresh, finely chopped cilantro

vegan chicken pieces, 1½ x the size and thickness of your palm

5 Little Gem lettuce leaves

½ ripe mango, chopped

10 cucumber ribbons

½ tsp sesame oil

3 cashew nuts, chopped

½ red chili, thinly sliced, to garnish

2–3 fresh mint leaves, torn, to garnish

This dish just makes me happy! Sesame and ginger partner amazingly, and the addition of mango really brightens up a dull day when you're in need of motivation. To make the zingy flavors of this Asian salad really sing, I recommend marinating the vegan chicken overnight in the fridge, or for at least 2 hours.

1 First, make the marinade. In a bowl, combine the lime zest and juice, sesame seeds, ginger, garlic, and cilantro and stir to mix well. Add the vegan chicken pieces and turn to coat thoroughly, then place in the fridge to marinate.

2 On a plate, arrange the baby gem leaves with the mango and cucumber ribbons.

3 Heat the sesame oil in a non-stick skillet over medium heat and fry the marinated vegan chicken pieces for 5 minutes, stirring frequently.

4 Spoon the Asian-flavored vegan chicken on top of the salad plate and garnish with chopped cashews, chili slices, and fresh torn mint.

IMPORTANT

This recipe is best when marinated overnight, so make sure you plan ahead with this meal.

MOROCCAN SPICED CAULIFLOWER

1 large cauliflower "steak"

1 tsp extra virgin olive oil

1 tsp cumin

1 tsp cinnamon

½ tsp paprika

1 tsp sumac

½ tsp white pepper

1 tbsp full-fat Greek yogurt OR Greek-style soy-based vegan yogurt

14.5oz (425g) can of green lentils

½ small red onion, finely chopped

small handful of fresh, finely chopped cilantro

small handful of fresh, finely chopped mint

small handful of fresh, finely chopped basil

zest and juice of 1 lime

2 tbsp pomegranate seeds

Whole cauliflower heads are great for slicing into thick "steaks," as they are delicious either roasted or grilled, and they can absorb all the flavors they are marinated in. They are also fat-free, cholesterol-free, and guilt-free, so enjoy!

1 Preheat the oven to 400°F.

2 Place the 1-inch-thick cauliflower steak in a mixing bowl, drizzle it with olive oil, and sprinkle the spices over it. Add the yogurt and turn the cauliflower in the marinade until it is thoroughly coated.

3 Transfer the steak onto a non-stick baking sheet and cook in the oven for 25 minutes until golden brown—the smell will be amazing!

4 While the steak is cooking, place the lentils in the same mixing bowl with the onion and chopped herbs and mix with the lime zest and juice and pomegranate seeds.

5 Serve the steak on a plate and spoon the tangy, herby lentil salad over the top.

CHICKEN AND MUSHROOM CACCIATORE

SERVES TWO

2 tsp extra virgin olive oil

½ red or white onion, finely sliced

1 garlic clove, crushed

4 closed cup mushrooms, sliced

7oz (200g) chopped tomatoes (½ x 14oz/400g) can

2 heaping tsp finely chopped rosemary, plus a little extra to garnish

2 chicken breast fillets, the size and thickness of your palm

handful of green beans

freshly ground black pepper

Cacciatore means "hunter" in Italian, so this is a classic hunter-style stew with a deliciously rich tomato sauce—exactly the kind of warming, healthy comfort food that I like.

1 Preheat the oven to 350°F.

2 Heat the oil in a non-stick saute pan over low heat and gently saute the onion and garlic until soft, around 4 minutes.

3 Add the mushrooms and saute for another 2 minutes, then add the chopped tomatoes and rosemary, stir, and gently simmer for 10 minutes, until thick.

4 Place the chicken breasts in an ovenproof dish and spoon the sauce over the top to cover. Bake in the oven for 20 minutes or until the chicken is cooked through.

5 Meanwhile, bring a pot of water to a boil and either boil or steam the green beans until done to your liking (see Good to Know, below).

6 Serve the chicken, topped with the rich sauce, alongside the green beans. Season with black pepper and garnish with a pinch of rosemary.

GOOD TO KNOW

Remember not to boil the life out of your vegetables—if you overcook them, they can get floppy and turn an olive-green color. Green beans should be a vibrant green color and have a crisp texture. Using a steamer to cook them conserves all the nutrients and keeps them a lovely bright green color.

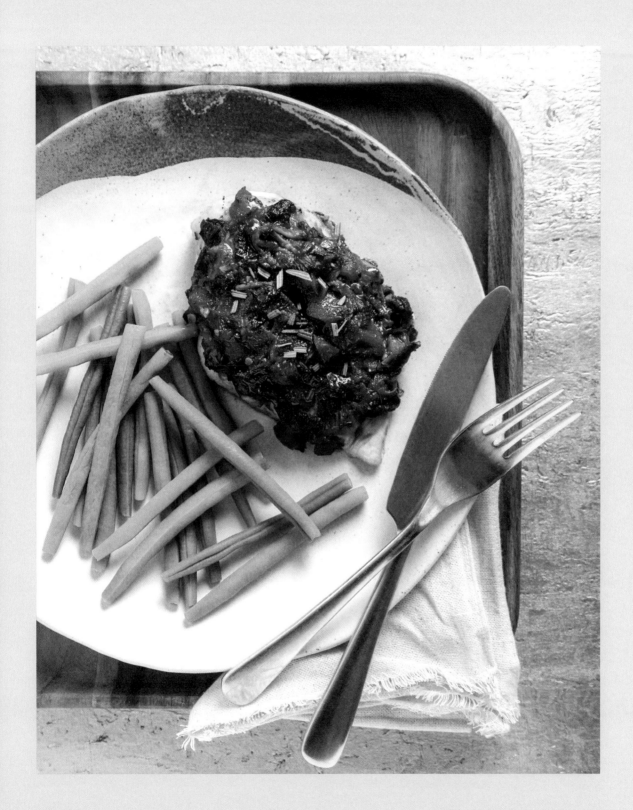

BUTTERBEAN STEW

SERVES ONE

1 tsp extra virgin olive oil

½ small red or white onion, finely chopped

1 garlic clove, crushed

2 white button mushrooms, chopped

½ tsp paprika

pinch of white pepper

1 heaping tsp fresh, finely chopped basil

7oz (200g) chopped tomatoes (½ x 14oz/400g) can

1 tsp tomato paste

pinch of dried chili flakes

1 heaping tsp finely chopped flat-leaf parsley

15.5oz (439g) can of butterbeans, drained and rinsed

handful of fresh spinach

squeeze of lemon

freshly ground black pepper

This lovely stew, with its rich tomato base and lemon and paprika flavors, reminds me of Spanish tapas. The addition of butterbeans allows you to stock up on some essential protein and B vitamins.

1 Heat the oil in a large non-stick saute pan over low to medium heat and gently saute the onion and garlic until soft. Add the mushrooms, paprika, white pepper, basil, tomatoes, tomato paste, chili flakes, and chopped parsley and stir together along with a generous ⅓ cup (100ml) water. Simmer for 5 minutes.

2 Add the butterbeans and simmer for another 5 minutes.

3 Stir in the spinach until wilted, add a squeeze of lemon, and season with black pepper.

4 Serve in your favorite dish and enjoy!

GOOD TO KNOW

I love the texture of large butterbeans, but you can use any type of canned beans for this dish—black beans or kidney beans, for example.

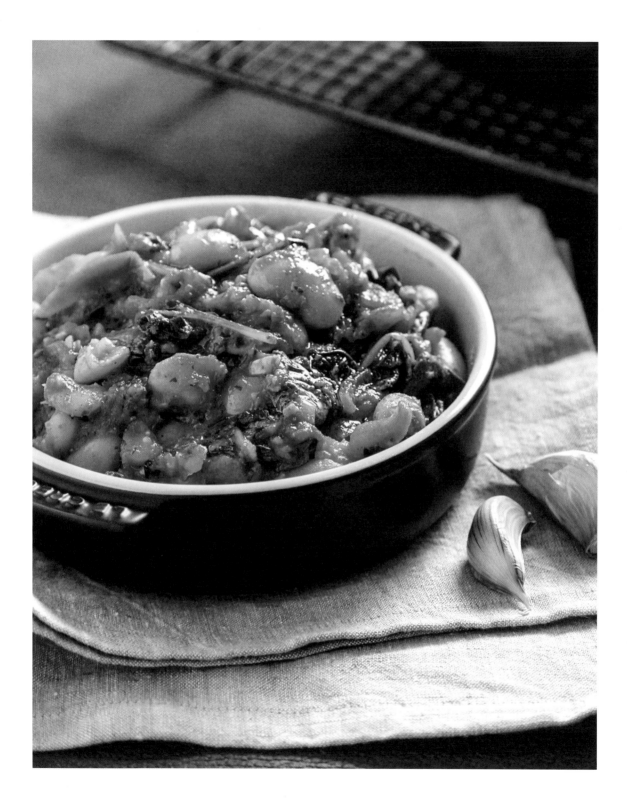

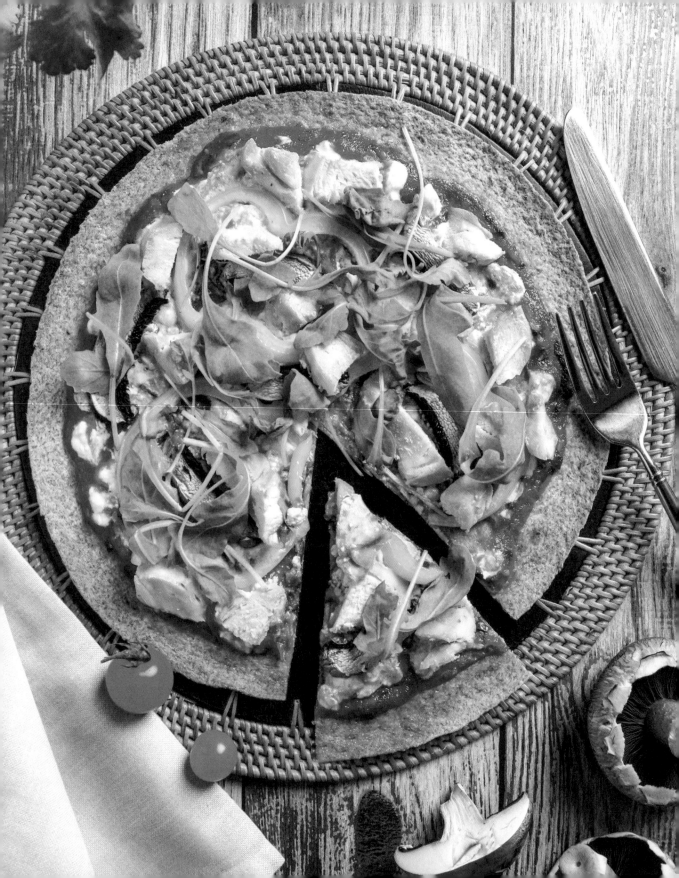

FULLY LOADED PIZZA

SERVES ONE

1 chicken breast, the size and thickness of your palm

1 whole-wheat wrap

1 tsp extra virgin olive oil

½ garlic clove, crushed

8 fresh basil leaves, finely chopped

1 tbsp tomato paste

1 tbsp full-fat cottage cheese

½ green (bell) pepper, thinly sliced

1 mushroom, thinly sliced

handful of arugula leaves

Ah, pizza! We all love it, and there are so many different kinds to choose... but they aren't always the healthiest of options! Therefore, I wanted to create something tasty and guilt-free —just pure enjoyment!

1 Preheat the oven to 350°F.

2 Place the chicken in an ovenproof dish and cook in the oven for 15–20 minutes. Set aside to cool.

3 Meanwhile, place the whole-wheat wrap on an oven or pizza tray and, using your fingers, massage the olive oil all over the top.

4 Place the garlic, basil, and tomato paste in a small bowl with a splash of water and mix well until you have a runny sauce. Spread this over the top of the wrap, leaving a border about an inch thick around the edge. Sprinkle the cottage cheese over the tomato sauce and top with the sliced pepper and mushroom.

5 Bake the pizza for 5 minutes. While it is cooking, shred the cooked chicken and then scatter this over the top of the pizza. Return the pizza to the oven for a final 5 minutes, then top with arugula leaves, slice into quarters, and serve.

COZZE ALLA MARINARA WITH FRIES

SERVES ONE

1 small sweet potato, sliced into chunky French fries

1 tsp extra virgin olive oil

2 tbsp tomato paste

1 red chili, finely chopped

2 garlic cloves, crushed

6 cherry tomatoes, quartered

2 tbsp finely chopped flat-leaf parsley, plus a little extra to garnish

35 mussels

freshly ground black pepper

This recipe brings a taste of Italy to your table. Mussels are a great source of lean protein, plus rich in key vitamins and minerals and heart-healthy omega-3 fats, and they're also a very sustainable choice of seafood. When I want to use potato in a recipe, I often choose sweet potato, as it is high in vitamins, antioxidants, and fiber. This is beyond delicious!

1 Preheat the oven to 400°F.

2 Toss the sweet potato fries in the olive oil and season with black pepper, then place on a baking sheet and bake for 20–30 minutes. If you like your fries a little softer, cook at a slightly lower heat.

3 Place a large non-stick pan with a lid over medium heat. Add the tomato paste, chili, and garlic and stir-fry quickly for about 30 seconds. Add a generous ⅓ cup (100ml) water and stir for a minute, then stir in the cherry tomatoes and parsley and cook for another minute.

4 Rinse the mussels, removing any sand or grit from the shells and pulling the "beards" from the shell to clean them.

5 Add the cleaned, fresh mussels to the pan. Give everything a good stir, then cover with the lid and let the mussels steam for 5–7 minutes, shaking the pan halfway through to make sure that all the mussel shells are opening and everything is coated in the delicious sauce.

6 Once you are ready to serve, it's important to check for unopened mussels and to dispose of any you find.

7 Serve the opened mussels in a large bowl, drizzle the sauce over them, and garnish with an extra pinch of parsley and a grind of black pepper.

GOOD TO KNOW

You can use the shell of a mussel like a pincer to remove the others.

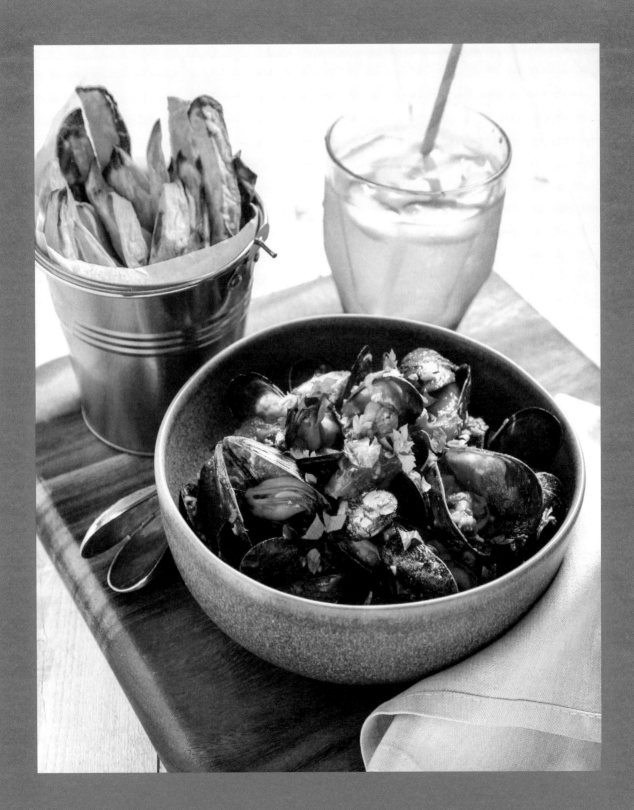

FABULOUS FALAFELS

SERVES 2 (Makes 12 falafel balls)

15oz (425g) can of chickpeas, drained and rinsed

7oz (200g) frozen broad beans, slightly defrosted

4 tbsp oats, pureed into a powder

1 garlic clove, crushed

1 tbsp sesame seeds

1 tbsp pumpkin seeds

½ tsp cumin

½ tsp cayenne pepper

pinch of white pepper

1 heaping tbsp fresh, finely chopped cilantro, plus a little extra to garnish

1 egg, beaten

2 tsp extra virgin olive oil

green, leafy salad, to serve

1 tbsp Raita (see p150) OR 1 tbsp full-fat Greek yogurt OR Greek-style soy-based vegan yogurt, per serving (optional)

FOR THE BABA GHANOUSH

1 small purple eggplant

juice of ½ lemon

1 small garlic clove, finely chopped

pinch of onion powder

pinch of ground cumin

pinch of chopped flat-leaf parsley

Falafels are delicious Middle Eastern balls of chickpea goodness. They are an excellent source of plant-based protein and full of fiber, plus all the antioxidant-rich spices pack such a flavor punch. They go perfectly with a smooth and silky baba ghanoush (also rich in protein and fiber), as the textures complement each other perfectly.

1 Preheat the oven to 350°F.

2 First, make the baba ghanoush. With a fork, prick the eggplant all over to ensure the steam can escape, then place on a wire rack and cook in the oven for 30 minutes. When cool enough to handle, scoop out the soft flesh and transfer to a blender with all the remaining ingredients and blend until you have the consistency you like.

3 Now, make the falafel. Place all the ingredients apart from the egg and the oil in a blender and blend on a low setting until you have a rough paste. Add the egg and blend to combine, then split the mixture into 12 equal portions and roll each one into a round falafel ball.

4 Heat 1 teaspoon of extra virgin olive oil in a non-stick skillet over medium heat and fry the falafels, turning continuously, for about 10 minutes. Add the remaining oil and fry for another 10 minutes, until they are all evenly browned and cooked through.

5 Sprinkle the falafels with a little chopped cilantro and serve with a green leafy salad and a tablespoon of baba ghanoush, raita, or Greek yogurt.

GOOD TO KNOW

Stored in an airtight container, the falafels will keep for 3 days. The baba ghanoush can also be stored in an airtight container and will keep in the fridge for a few days. Alternatively, you can freeze it in freezer bags, and it will keep for up to a month

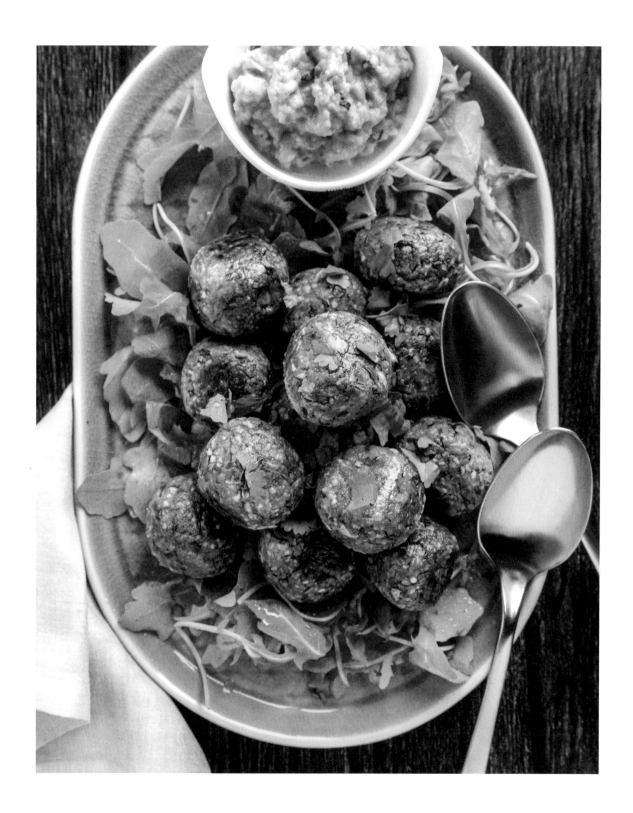

FISH STEW

1 tsp extra virgin olive oil

1 garlic clove, crushed

½ small white or red onion, roughly chopped

handful of finely chopped flat-leaf parsley, plus extra to garnish

14oz (400g) can of chopped tomatoes

6 black olives, sliced

2 cod fillets, each the size and thickness of your palm

freshly ground black pepper

handful of fresh spinach

2 wedges of lemon

This recipe is not only quick and easy to make, it's also full of goodness. The white fish is a great source of lean protein, the olives are full of heart-healthy monounsaturated fat, and the spinach contributes lots of iron and fiber—it's an all-around winner!

1 Preheat the oven to 350°F.

2 Heat the olive oil in a large non-stick saute pan over medium-low heat and gently saute the garlic and onion until soft.

3 Transfer the garlic and onion to an ovenproof dish and mix in the chopped parsley, tomatoes, and sliced olives. Add the cod fillets and ensure they are entirely covered with the sauce. Season generously with black pepper, then bake in the oven for 15 minutes.

4 Stir the spinach into the sauce, then return the dish to the oven for a final 5 minutes.

5 Divide the cod between two plates, garnish with a sprig of fresh parsley, and serve with a wedge of lemon.

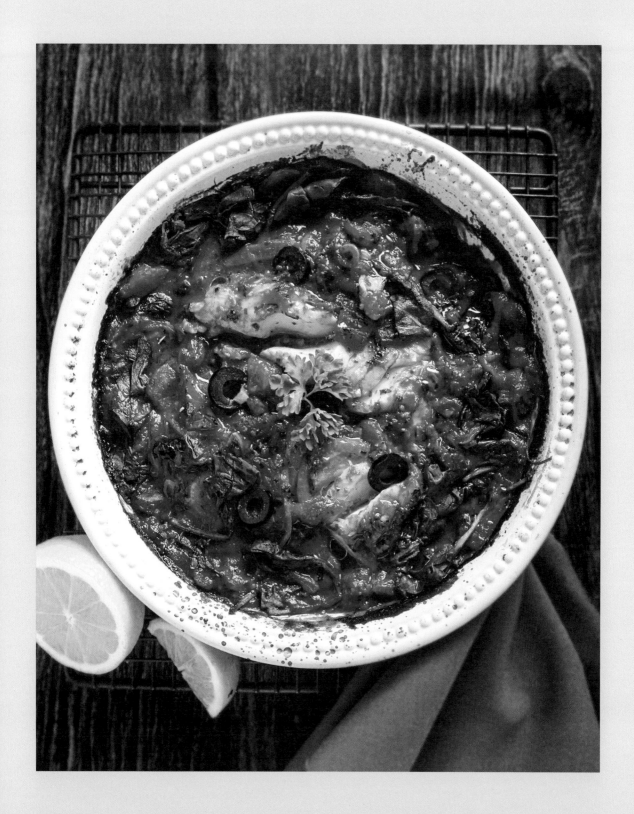

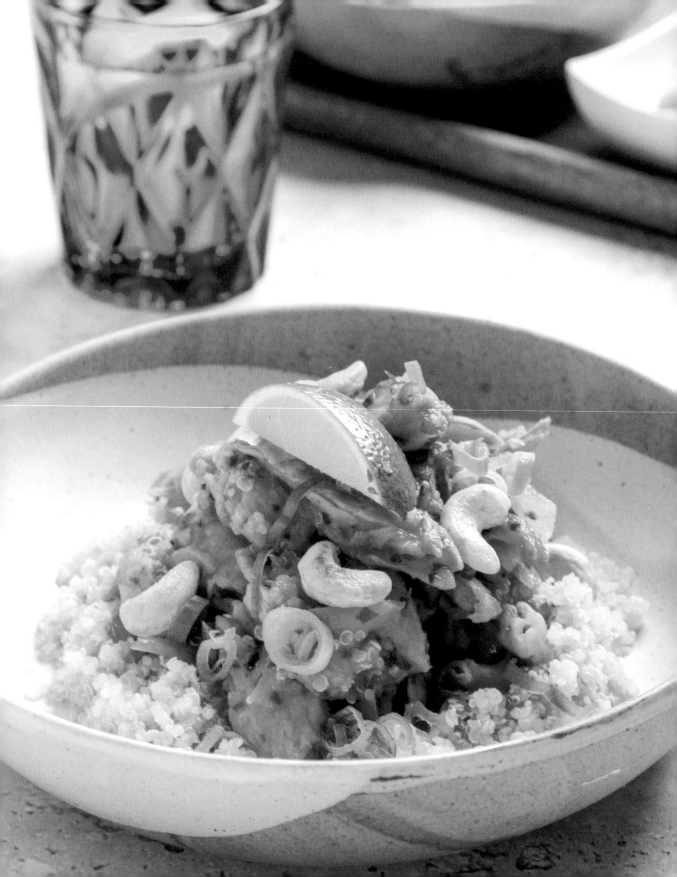

SWEET AND SOUR

handful of chopped pineapple

1 thumb-size piece of fresh ginger root

½ small red chili, chopped

2 garlic cloves, chopped

1 tomato, chopped

1 tsp tomato paste

1 stick of lemongrass

handful of fresh, finely chopped cilantro

juice of ½ lime

2 lime leaves

vegan chicken pieces, 3 x the size and thickness of your palm

handful of chopped red or green pepper

handful of chopped red onion

12 cashew nuts

1¾oz (50g) quinoa (150g cooked weight)

1 green onion, finely sliced

wedge of lime, to serve

This is another healthy spin on a takeout favorite that contains all the popular piquant flavors but none of the nasty ones. Just what you need on a weekend night—quick, fresh, wholesome food with tons of flavor.

1 Start by making the sweet and sour sauce. In a blender, add the pineapple, ginger, red chili, garlic, tomato, and tomato paste with a scant 1 cup (200ml) water. Puree to a smooth consistency.

2 Transfer the sauce to a medium saucepan. Hit the lemongrass stick to release its flavor and then add to the pan with the cilantro, lime juice, and lime leaves. Bring to a boil, then reduce the heat and simmer for 5 minutes.

3 Add the vegan chicken, pepper, and onion to the pan and simmer for 10 minutes to allow the vegetables to soften.

4 Now, toast the cashew nuts. Place a dry pan over low heat and gently toast the cashews for 2–3 minutes, until golden.

5 Bring a saucepan of water to a boil and cook the quinoa according to the package instructions, then drain.

6 Divide the cooked quinoa between serving bowls and top with the sweet and sour chicken. Garnish with a scattering of green onion and toasted cashews and serve with a wedge of lime.

PAN-FRIED SEA BASS WITH GARLIC AND CHILI

SERVES TWO

2 tsp extra virgin olive oil

1 red pepper, sliced

1 large zucchini, sliced

1 large red onion, sliced

2 sea bass fillets, the size and thickness of your palm

pinch of chili flakes

1 small garlic clove, finely chopped

pinch of fresh, finely chopped cilantro, to garnish

wedge of lemon

I like sea bass but you can choose freshwater bass if you prefer. Like most white fish, bass is an excellent source of protein, and it tastes great with the chili, garlic, and this medley of Italian-style vegetables.

1 Heat half of the olive oil in a skillet over medium heat and stir-fry all the vegetables until they are cooked to your liking. Transfer to a dish, cover to keep warm, and set aside.

2 Return the pan to low heat with the remaining olive oil and add the sea bass fillets. Season with half the chili and garlic and cook for approximately 10 minutes, until lightly browned and cooked through. Gently turn the fish with a spatula, scatter the remaining chili and garlic over it, and cook until this side is also lightly browned.

3 Divide the vegetables between two serving plates and place a sea bass fillet on top. Garnish with cilantro and serve with a wedge of lemon for squeezing.

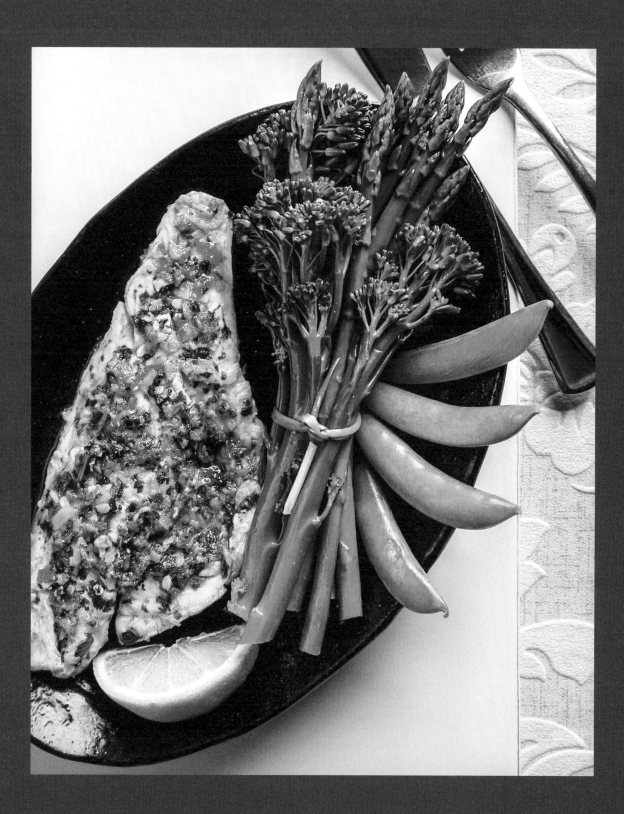

SWEET POTATO AND COCONUT CURRY

SERVES TWO

2 handfuls of diced sweet potato

1 tsp coconut oil

½ red onion, finely chopped

2 garlic cloves, finely chopped

pinch of chili flakes

high-protein meat alternative, 3 x the size and thickness of your palm

1 tsp fennel seeds

1 tsp ground cumin

1 tsp garam masala

¼ tsp white pepper

2 tbsp coconut milk

small handful of fresh spinach

juice of ½ lemon

pinch of dried, shredded coconut

small handful of fresh, finely chopped cilantro

½ red chili, finely chopped (optional)

This dish is perfect for a super-quick supper and can even be reheated or eaten cold for lunch on the go. I love using a plant-based meat alternative, as the texture is perfect for absorbing all the delicious flavors. Spinach makes the dish feel authentically Indian and adds a nice color and a good nutritional hit.

1 Bring a pan of water to a boil and cook the sweet potato for around 15 minutes until soft, then drain and set aside.

2 While your sweet potatoes are boiling, you can quickly prepare the rest of the dish. Heat the coconut oil in a non-stick saute pan over low heat and cook the onion until it caramelizes—this slow cooking will allow it to release all its sweetness. Add the garlic and chili flakes and cook for another minute.

3 Add the meat alternative along with all the spices and stir until everything is coated. Add the cooked sweet potato to the pan with 3½ tablespoons water, bring to a simmer, and cook for 5 minutes.

4 Add the coconut milk and spinach and wait for the spinach to wilt slightly, then stir in the lemon juice. Serve in a bowl, garnished with the dried coconut, freshly chopped cilantro, and a little chili if you like extra heat!

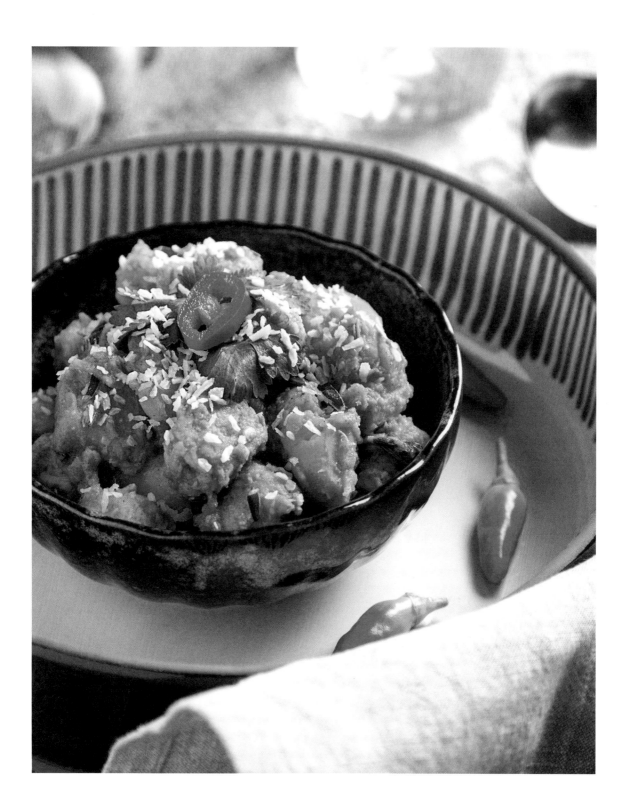

SALMON AND BOK CHOI WITH GINGER AND GARLIC

1 garlic clove, finely chopped

1 tsp grated fresh ginger root

½ fresh red chili, finely chopped

1 salmon fillet, the size and thickness of your palm

1 tsp black sesame seeds

handful of baby bok choi

1 tsp sesame oil

This dish is so easy to make but packed full of goodness. The bok choi is full of fiber, vitamins, minerals, and antioxidants, and I like to cook it so that it retains a slight crunch. Black sesame seeds, unlike white, are still in their hull, which means they have a little more texture and certainly more nutritional value.

1 Preheat the oven to 350°F.

2 First, make the marinade. In a bowl, mix the garlic, ginger, and chili together.

3 Coat the salmon with half the marinade mixture, sprinkle with black sesame seeds, and place on a non-stick baking sheet. Cook in the oven for 15 minutes, or until cooked.

4 Coat the bok choi in the remaining marinade and, 5 minutes before the salmon is ready, heat the sesame oil in a non-stick saute pan. Add the bok choi to the pan and saute for 5 minutes.

5 Arrange the salmon and bok choi on a plate and enjoy!

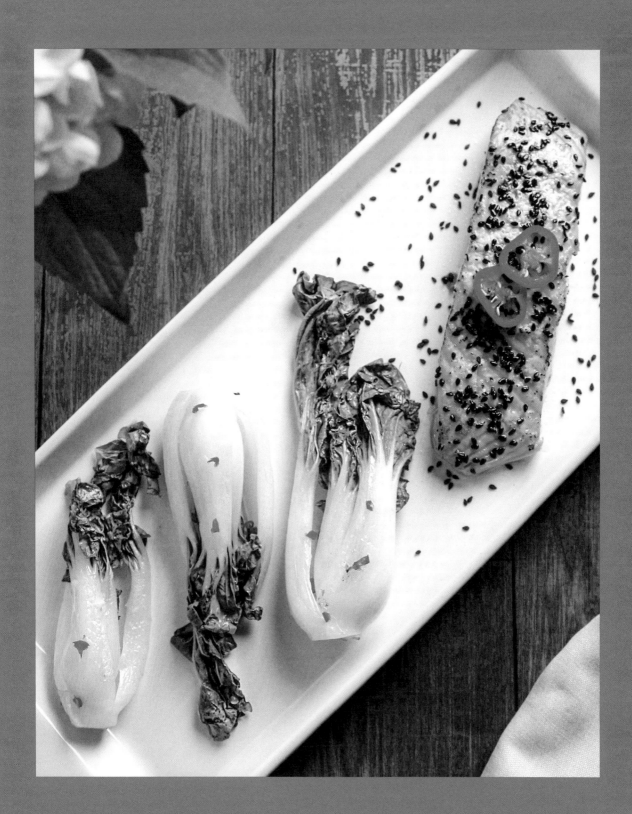

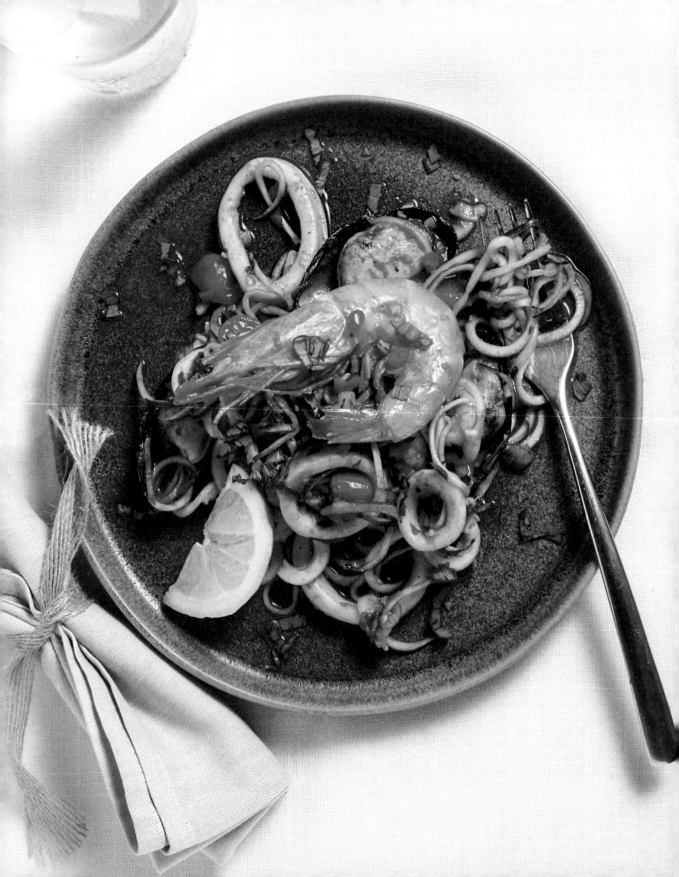

FRUITS DE LA MARE

SERVES ONE

1 tsp extra virgin olive oil

2 tbsp tomato paste

1 red chili, chopped

2 garlic cloves, finely chopped

6 cherry tomatoes, quartered

small handful of finely chopped flat-leaf parsley, plus a little extra to garnish

large handful of mixed seafood, fresh or frozen

big handful of zucchini noodles (spiralized zucchini)

freshly ground black pepper

wedge of lemon, to serve

This is one of my favorite "go-to" meals. It literally takes 10 minutes or so to cook from start to finish, it's bursting with flavor, and the seafood delivers essential vitamins, minerals, and heart-healthy omega-3 fats.

1 Heat the olive oil in a non-stick pan over medium heat. Add the tomato paste, chili, and garlic and stir-fry quickly for about 30 seconds. Add a generous ⅓ cup (100ml) water and stir for a minute, then stir in the cherry tomatoes and parsley and cook for another minute.

2 Add the seafood, mixing it thoroughly with the sauce, and cook for 7–10 minutes, or until cooked through.

3 Turn off the heat, add the zucchini noodles, and toss to combine. Season with more black pepper, garnish with fresh parsley, and serve with a nice wedge of lemon. Enjoy!

GOOD TO KNOW

Frozen seafood works very well for this recipe, but ensure it is completely defrosted before you use it.

OSTRICH STEAK, FRIES AND PEAS

1 small sweet potato, peeled and cut into French fries

1 tsp extra virgin olive oil

freshly ground black pepper

1 ostrich fillet, the size and thickness of your palm

2 white button mushrooms, finely sliced

1 large tomato, sliced in half

small handful of fresh or frozen peas

2 sprigs of flat-leaf parsley, finely chopped (optional)

This is steak and French fries, but not as you know it! It tastes as delicious as lean beef but, because it has none of the fat marbling, it is lower in calories, fat, and cholesterol. It's gaining in popularity, so it should be available at a supermarket near you or online. You can substitute bison or another lean exotic meat if you can't find ostrich.

1 Preheat the oven to 350°F.

2 Place the sweet potato chips in a roasting pan, toss in the olive oil, and season with black pepper. Place in the oven for approximately 30 minutes, until lightly browned and cooked through. A crispier version can be achieved by baking them at a slightly higher temperature (400°F).

3 Place a non-stick saute pan over medium heat and dry saute the ostrich steak for 3–4 minutes on each side, depending on the thickness (take care not to overcook—see Good to Know). Remove from heat, transfer to a plate, cover, and leave to rest.

4 Meanwhile, return the non-stick pan to the heat and stir-fry the mushrooms in the meat juices for 3–4 minutes. Arrange the tomatoes in an ovenproof dish and place under a hot broiler for 3–4 minutes. Bring a pan of water to a boil and cook the peas for 3–5 minutes.

5 Serve all the ingredients on a plate, garnished with fresh parsley, if you like.

GOOD TO KNOW

It's important not to cook the lean steak past rare to medium-rare, as it will continue to cook after it has been removed from the heat source. It is also crucial to allow it to rest as, during this time, it reabsorbs the juices that would otherwise be lost. When you cut the meat and taste it, you will notice it is juicier and tastier.

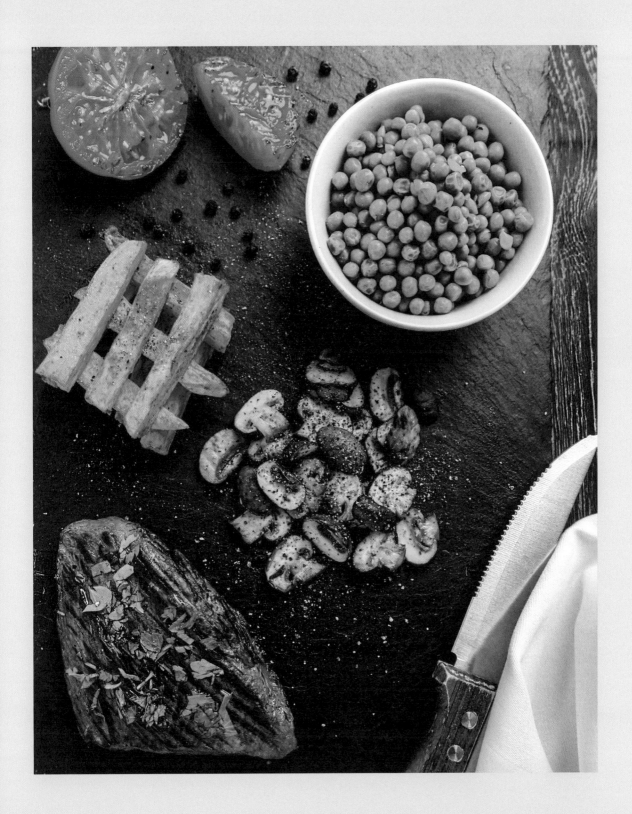

TURKEY FAJITAS

SERVES TWO

1 tbsp Smashed Avocado (see p48)

1 red pepper, cut into thin strips

turkey breasts, 2 x the size and thickness of your palm, cut into small strips

juice of ½ lemon

2 whole-wheat tortillas

FOR THE RUB

1 garlic clove, crushed

½ tsp white pepper

½ tsp paprika

½ tsp allspice

pinch cayenne pepper

1 tsp Italian seasoning

1 tsp extra virgin olive oil

Turkey fajitas are fun to make with the whole family, and this tasty Mexican dish is packed with protein and vitamins. It's the citrus flavors—the lemon with the turkey and the lime in the smashed avocado—that really stand out in this recipe, so don't hold back.

1 First, make the smashed avocado (p48) and keep in the fridge until you are ready to serve it.

2 Place a non-stick saute pan over low-to-medium heat and saute the pepper for 10 minutes.

3 Meanwhile, make the rub. Place all the ingredients in a bowl and mix together. Add the turkey strips and turn them over in the rub, massaging the flavors in with your hands, if you like, until thoroughly coated.

4 Add the turkey to the pan with the pepper, turn up the heat, and pour in ⅓ cup (75ml) water. Bring to a simmer, then turn down the heat and cook until the liquid starts to evaporate. You want the turkey to be cooked through and a little juice left in the pan.

5 Squeeze the lemon juice over the top and give everything in the pan a good stir.

6 Quickly heat the tortillas using either a microwave or, as I prefer, in a dry skillet over a gas burner, turning them frequently to prevent burning.

7 To serve, spread the smashed avocado over the warmed tortilla, top with some spicy turkey fajitas and peppers, then wrap them up and enjoy all the delicious flavors!

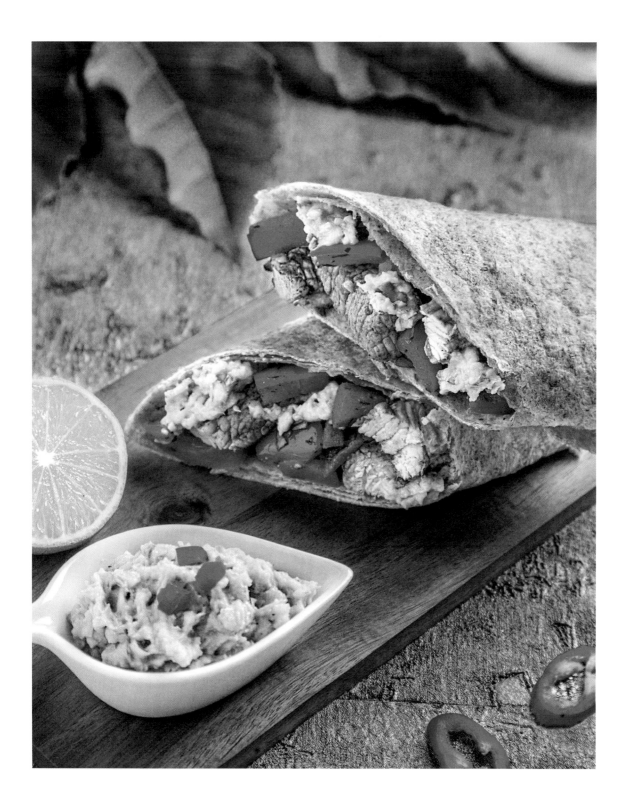

LOADED NACHOS

SERVES TWO

2 tsp extra virgin olive oil

½ white or red onion, finely chopped

1 red chili, finely chopped

1 yellow pepper, finely chopped

2 garlic cloves, finely chopped

1 tsp ground cumin

½ tsp ground cinnamon

½ tsp cayenne pepper

2 x 15.5oz (439g) cans of mixed beans (kidney, pinto, cannellini —all are good), drained and rinsed

2 tbsp tomato paste

bunch of fresh cilantro, finely chopped

2 sweet potato wraps

Making nachos from sweet potato wraps means they're gluten-free, high in fiber, and low in calories, as well as crispy and crunchy and perfect for loading! I always keep cans of beans in the pantry, as they're such a great source of plant protein. However, it's important to look for brands with "no added sugar" and that are "low sodium." I do rinse mine with water over a bowl to reduce the sodium content even more.

1 Preheat the oven to 400°F and line a baking sheet with parchment paper.

2 Heat the oil in a non-stick saute pan over medium heat and cook the onion, chili, and pepper for 4–5 minutes, until they are soft and caramelized. Add the garlic and cook, stirring, for a further minute. Add the spices to the pan and cook until fragrant, then add the beans and stir to coat.

3 Add the tomato paste with 5 tablespoons of water and bring to a boil, then reduce to a simmer and cook for around 10 minutes.

4 Add a good handful of chopped cilantro. Reserve a little for a garnish, but do be generous, as this ingredient really makes the dish.

5 Now, make the nachos. Cut the wraps into small triangle shapes and spread over the baking sheet. Bake in your oven for just 5 minutes, turning halfway through.

6 Once the nachos are nice and crispy, serve the chili in a bowl topped with the remaining cilantro, then add the nachos ready for loading!

GOOD TO KNOW

If you like spice, sprinkle the sweet potato wraps with some chili powder before you crisp them up in the oven!

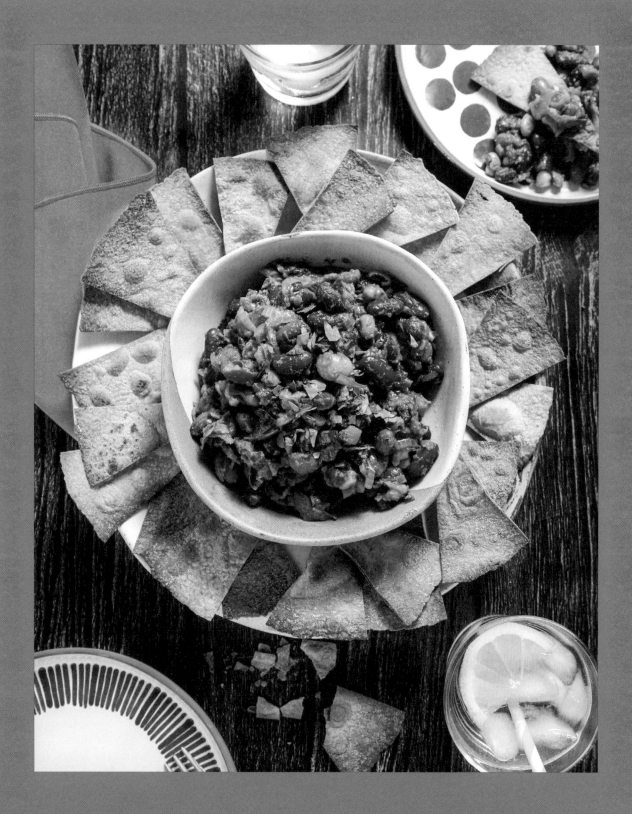

CHICKEN SATAY SPECIAL

chicken breast, the size and thickness of your palm, cut into large cubes

handful of mixed peppers, cut into large cubes (big enough to skewer)

1 tsp all-natural peanut butter

¼ tsp grated fresh ginger root

juice of ¼ lime

pinch of cayenne pepper

sprinkle of fresh, finely chopped cilantro, to garnish

1 green onion, finely chopped, to garnish

This delicious combo of chicken and peanut butter packs a powerful protein punch. Just remember to pick the best quality, all-natural peanut butter you can find (one without added sugars and oils) in order to achieve that authentic satay flavor!

1 Preheat the broiler. Adjust the rack to midway in the oven.

2 Thread the chicken and pepper cubes alternately onto a large skewer, then place under the broiler and cook, turning frequently, for approximately 15 minutes, until cooked through.

3 While the chicken is cooking, make the satay sauce. Place a non-stick saute pan over low heat, add the peanut butter, ginger, lime juice, and cayenne pepper, and stir together until the peanut butter has softened. Add a splash of water if necessary—you need the right consistency for drizzling.

4 Arrange the chicken and red pepper skewer on your favorite plate and then drizzle it with the satay sauce. Garnish with chopped cilantro and green onion, and enjoy.

SWEET POTATO KORMA

1 tsp flaxseed oil

½ white onion, finely chopped

1 green chili, finely chopped

1 tsp cumin

½ tsp turmeric

1 cardamom pod, crushed

½ thumb-size piece of ginger, finely chopped

1 garlic clove, finely chopped

handful of diced sweet potato

vegan chicken pieces, 3 x the size and thickness of your palm

2 tsp tomato paste

1¾oz (50g) dry buckwheat (4¼oz/120g cooked weight)

1 tsp poppy seeds

small handful of fresh, finely chopped cilantro

1 tbsp flaked almonds

1 tbsp full-fat Greek yogurt OR Greek-style soy-based vegan yogurt

This vegan curry is a delicate, creamy, and nutty delight. Serving it with buckwheat instead of white rice really raises the bar nutritionally, and the poppy seeds and almonds provide even more healthy fats, fiber, and essential nutrients, along with a welcome crunch.

1 Warm the flaxseed oil in a medium saucepan over medium heat and gently saute the onion with the green chili and dry spices for around 3 minutes. Add the ginger and garlic and saute for another minute so they release their flavors.

2 Add the sweet potato, vegan chicken, and tomato paste along with 1¾ cups (400ml) water and bring to a boil. Once boiling, reduce to a simmer, and cook for 10 minutes, or until the sweet potato is cooked through.

3 Meanwhile, bring a pot of water to a boil and prepare the buckwheat according to the package instructions, about 15 minutes. Strain and place in a mixing bowl. Add the poppy seeds and half the chopped cilantro and stir thoroughly, then cover and set aside.

4 In a skillet over medium heat, saute the flaked almonds for 2 minutes until they are nicely toasted and golden. Set aside.

5 Once the sweet potato is cooked through, take the pan off the heat and stir in the yogurt.

6 To serve, divide the buckwheat between two bowls, spoon over the korma, and garnish with the remaining chopped cilantro and toasted almonds.

FEAST FROM THE EAST

1 x 15oz (425g) can of chickpeas, drained and rinsed

1 tsp ras el hanout

1 tsp extra virgin olive oil

½ red pepper, chopped

½ green pepper, chopped

3 tbsp full-fat Greek yogurt OR Greek-style soy-based vegan yogurt

a few fresh mint leaves, chopped, plus a little extra to garnish

squeeze of lemon

This wonderfully fragrant dish is so simple to make, as the ras el hanout spice mix does all the heavy lifting. It's an earthy mix of many spices that generally includes cardamom, nutmeg, anise, mace, cinnamon, ginger, various peppercorns, and turmeric, but the breadth and variety are endlessly versatile. Do add it to your shelf of go-to spices.

1 Preheat the oven to 400°F.

2 Pour the rinsed chickpeas onto a clean paper towel to dry, then transfer them to a baking sheet with the ras el hanout and toss until they are all thoroughly coated. Roast for 30–40 minutes until nice and crunchy, turning occasionally, then set aside to cool.

3 Meanwhile, place the oil in a non-stick saute pan over low heat and gently saute the peppers until slightly soft and starting to caramelize.

4 In a bowl, mix the crunchy spiced chickpeas with the peppers and the remaining ingredients, then serve with an extra sprig of fresh mint.

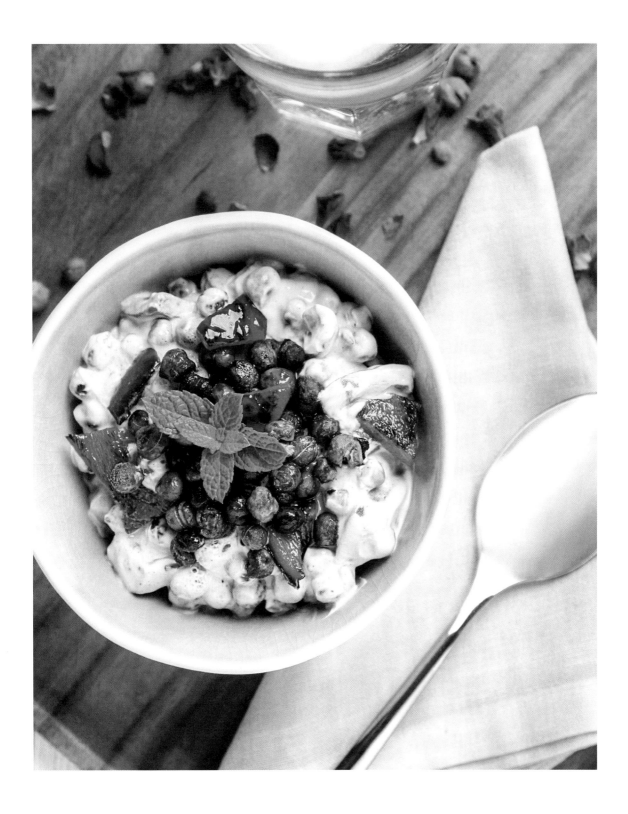

MALDIVIAN WRAP

SERVES TWO

canned tuna in spring water
(2 x the size and thickness of
your palm), drained

1 tsp dried, shredded coconut

1 red chili, deseeded and finely
sliced

freshly ground black pepper

2 sweet potato or whole-wheat
wraps

2 small tomatoes, sliced

½ small red onion, sliced

1 avocado, sliced

2 lime wedges

small handful of fresh, finely
chopped cilantro

The Maldives has got to be one of my favorite places. I was inspired to create this dish after enjoying their traditional breakfast, called mas huni. It's a very simple mix of tuna, onion, coconut, and chili, but everything is very finely chopped, and all the flavors are so tasty together!

1 Place the tuna in a bowl, mix with the coconut and chili, and season with freshly ground black pepper.

2 Heat the wraps—either in a warm oven for 5 minutes or toasted in a hot pan until beginning to brown.

3 Place the wraps on a plate and divide the tuna mixture between them. Top with the tomatoes, onion, and avocado, but be careful not to overfill, as otherwise the wraps will fall apart.

4 Squeeze the lime juice over the wraps (to taste) and sprinkle with cilantro.

CORONATION "CHICKEN" WRAP

SERVES TWO

½ tbsp plain sugar-free yogurt OR soy-based vegan yogurt

½ tsp curry powder

¼ tsp ground cinnamon

pinch of white pepper

1 tsp flaked almonds

2 tsp golden raisins

1 tsp extra virgin olive oil

high-protein meat alternative, 3 x the size and thickness of your palm

2 whole-wheat wraps

2 Little Gem lettuce leaves

1 medium tomato, sliced

1 heaping tsp fresh, finely chopped cilantro

This is a delectable twist on the British classic. Perfect for lunch on the go or a great addition to your summer picnic! And, if you have any left over, the lightly curried meat alternative makes an excellent filling in a baked sweet potato (see p54).

1 First, make the Coronation sauce. Place the yogurt, curry powder, cinnamon, and white pepper in a large bowl.

2 With a pestle and mortar, crush the almond flakes, then add to the bowl with the golden raisins and stir to combine.

3 In a saute pan, heat the extra virgin olive oil and stir-fry the high-protein meat alternative pieces on low to medium heat for about 10 minutes, or until it starts to brown nicely, then set aside to cool.

4 Heat the whole-wheat wraps—either in a warm oven for 5 minutes or toasted in a hot pan until beginning to brown.

5 Add the cooled "meat" to the Coronation sauce and stir to coat, then layer the wraps with lettuce leaves, Coronation meat alternative, and tomato slices, and dress with a sprinkling of cilantro.

LARGE SHRIMP COCKTAIL

SERVES ONE

4¼oz (120g) cooked large shrimp (peeled and deveined)

handful of shredded Little Gem lettuce

2 cherry tomatoes, quartered

½ avocado

pinch of paprika, to garnish

sprig of parsley, finely chopped, to garnish

wedge of lemon, to serve

FOR THE MARIE ROSE SAUCE

1 tbsp full-fat Greek yogurt OR Greek-style soy-based vegan yogurt

1 heaping tsp tomato paste

pinch of paprika

squeeze of lemon juice

Do you have a soft spot for a retro classic? Well, I do, and to me, this dish is a classic, an icon! However, of course, I've swapped the original mayonnaise for the much healthier Greek yogurt and added avocado (shrimp's perfect partner) to bring this dish into the 21st century!

1 First, make the sauce. In a bowl, mix the Greek yogurt, tomato sauce, paprika, and lemon juice until it turns a flamingo pink color. Add the cooked and peeled shrimp and turn them in the sauce to coat.

2 Take a stemmed glass and create layers with all your ingredients —the shrimp, lettuce, tomato, and avocado. Garnish the top of the glass with a sprinkle of paprika and parsley and serve with a wedge of lemon. In my opinion, though, hanging a shrimp off the edge of the glass is taking retro a step too far!

GOOD TO KNOW

Not sure how to devein a fresh shrimp? Just make a small slice down the middle of the back to expose the dark vein and pull—it should come out easily.

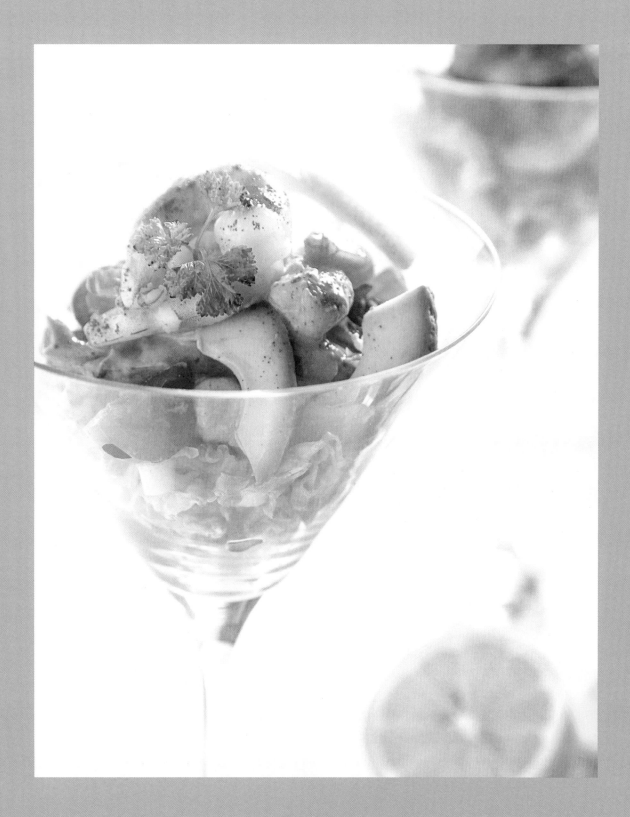

HAWAIIAN VEGAN PIZZA

SERVES ONE

1 whole-wheat wrap

1 tsp extra virgin olive oil

1 tbsp tomato paste

½ garlic clove, crushed

8 fresh basil leaves, finely chopped

vegan chicken pieces, 1½ x the size and thickness of your palm

1 pineapple slice, cut into small cubes

1 shallot, finely chopped

1 tsp dried oregano

Many people will tell you that pineapple shouldn't be on a pizza. However, don't let that stop you from trying this taste sensation! Whether you're vegan or not, I guarantee this pizza topping will be one you will come back to time and time again.

1 Preheat the oven to 400°F.

2 Place the whole-wheat wrap on an oven tray and drizzle all over with the olive oil, using your hands to spread it evenly over the surface.

3 In a small dish, mix the tomato paste, garlic, and basil with a splash of water to create a runny sauce, then spread this evenly over the wrap, leaving a ½in (1cm) border.

4 Scatter the vegan chicken and pineapple over the pizza base along with the shallot and oregano.

5 Bake in the oven for approximately 10 minutes, until the base has turned crispy. Enjoy!

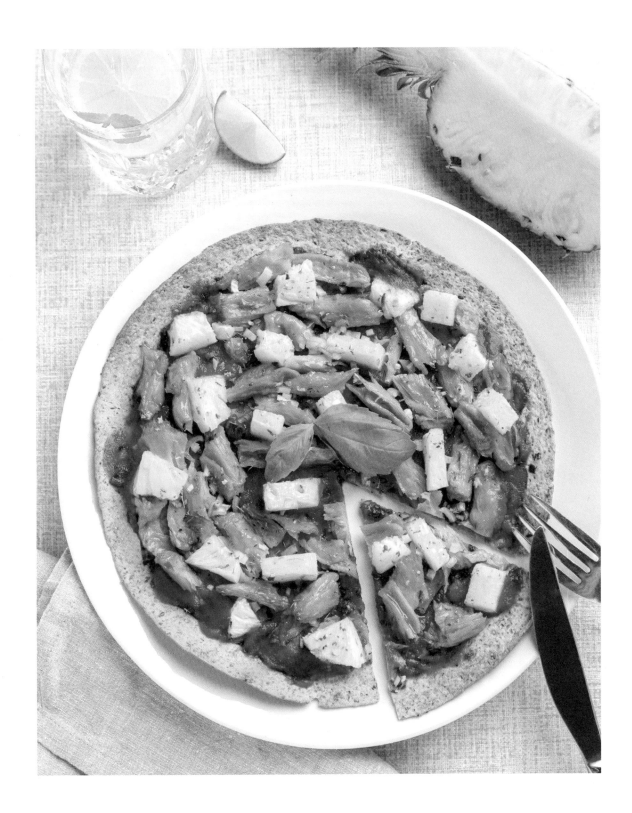

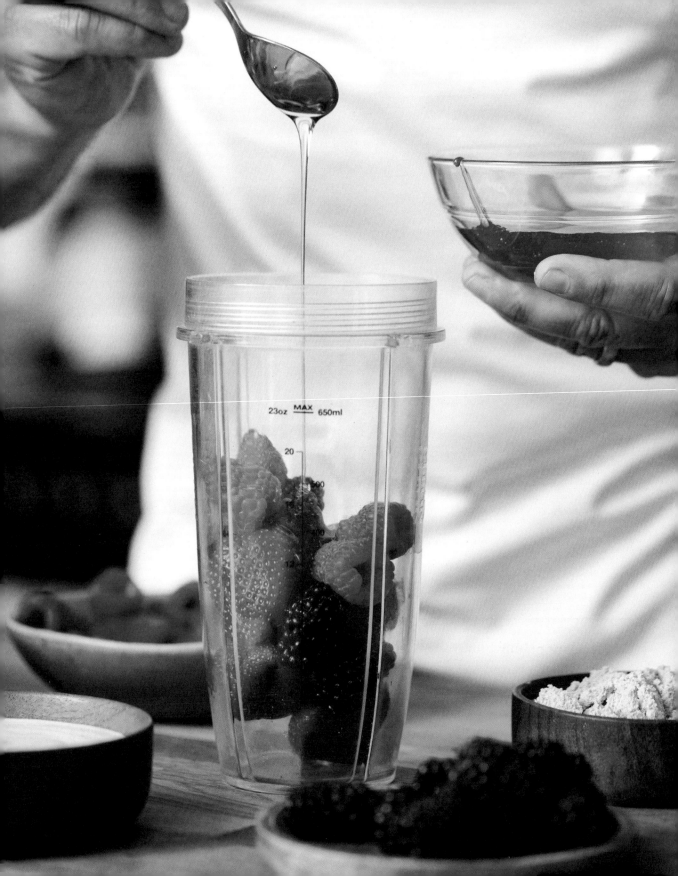

23oz MAX 650ml

20

16

12

These wonderfully healthy snacks are designed to keep you satiated and on track. They are also so simple to make and will show you just how delicious and indulgent healthy options can be.

SNACKS

LATTE LOVERS' PROTEIN SHAKE

SERVES ONE

½ cup strong coffee OR 1 single espresso coffee

1 tbsp rolled oats

½ serving (1 scoop/40ml) of The Six Pack Revolution Vanilla Caramel Heaven Post Workout Smoothie

scant 1 cup (200ml) unsweetened soy milk OR unsweetened pea milk

handful of ice cubes (optional)

dusting of ground cinnamon (optional)

This is the perfect way to perk up your morning—I only ever make it with good strong coffee to give me the lift I need, and, well, it just tastes better. The cinnamon is optional, but I highly recommend it, as it is both rich in antioxidants and believed to boost the metabolism.

1 First, make the coffee, then allow to cool.

2 Place the oats, protein powder, and soy milk in a blender. Add the coffee with a handful of ice (if using) and blend until smooth.

3 Pour into your favorite glass and top with a little cinnamon, if you like a bit of spice!

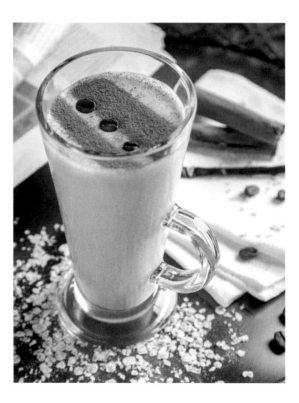

GOOD TO KNOW

This will count towards your caffeine quota for the day so cut back on that mid-morning coffee—replace it with herbal tea.

GREEN GODDESS SMOOTHIE

SERVES ONE

a few pieces of frozen sliced banana

a few pieces of frozen sliced pineapple

handful of fresh spinach leaves

2 tbsp full-fat Greek yogurt OR Greek-style soy-based vegan yogurt

scant 1 cup (200ml) unsweetened soy milk OR unsweetened pea milk

8 pistachios

1 tsp milled flaxseed

handful of ice cubes (optional)

This smoothie is not only delightfully sweet but also fiber-rich, which improves digestion and creates a feeling of satiety. Flaxseeds and pistachios are also high in heart-healthy fats, which can lower levels of bad cholesterol.

1 Place all the ingredients in a blender and blend until smooth, then pour into your favorite glass and enjoy.

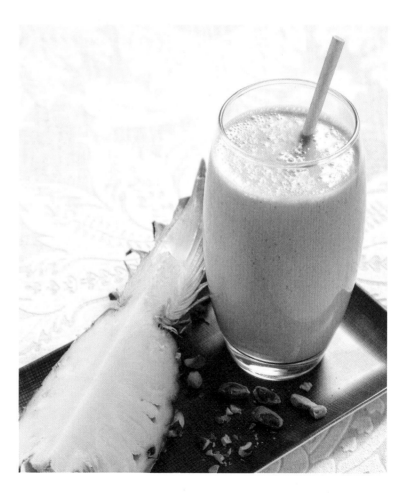

GOOD TO KNOW

You can use fresh instead of frozen banana and pineapple — it just won't be as cold.

WAKE-UP SMOOTHIE BOWL

SERVES ONE

½ serving (1 scoop/40ml) of The
Six Pack Vanilla Caramel Heaven
Post Workout Smoothie

1 frozen banana

scant 1 cup (200ml) unsweetened
almond milk OR water

1 tsp instant coffee granules

handful of fresh spinach

6 pecan halves, crushed

handful of ice cubes (optional)

This bowl of goodness "springs you to life," setting you up for the best day. Bonus... the pecans alone contain more than 19 vitamins and minerals, and you can choose between a rich caramel or decadent chocolate wake-up call (see Tip)!

1 Pick your preferred smoothie and place in a blender with all the remaining ingredients, apart from the pecans. Blend until smooth —for a lighter consistency, you can add a little more almond milk or water.

2 Pour the smoothie mixture into a bowl and sprinkle the crushed pecans over the top.

GOOD TO KNOW

You can swap the Vanilla Caramel Heaven Smoothie for The Six Pack Decadent Chocolate Caramel Post Workout Smoothie —it's equally delicious.

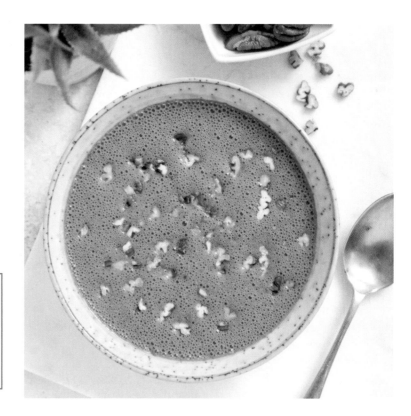

PIÑA COLADA SMOOTHIE

SERVES ONE

handful of frozen pineapple

3 tbsp full-fat Greek yogurt
OR Greek-style soy-based
vegan yogurt

scant 1 cup (200ml) coconut milk

2 tsp dried, shredded coconut

small handful of ice

This being my favorite cocktail, it was only a matter of time before it landed in my collection of recipes. I love the creamy coconut with the fruity pineapple—a match made in heaven!

1 Place all the ingredients in a blender and blend until smooth, then pour into your favorite glass and enjoy.

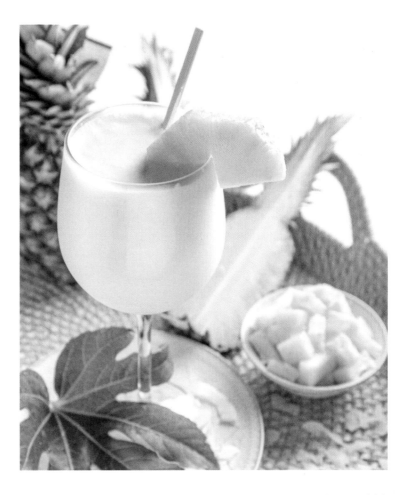

CARROT CAKE SHAKE

SERVES ONE

½ large orange, peeled and segmented (fresh or frozen)

½ banana, sliced (fresh or frozen)

2 tsp dried, shredded coconut

6 pecan halves, chopped

½ medium carrot, grated

2 tbsp full-fat Greek yogurt OR OR Greek-style soy-based vegan yogurt

scant 1 cup (200ml) unsweetened soy milk

½ tsp ground cinnamon

small handful of ice cubes (optional)

This shake is thick and creamy and tastes just like a slice of one of my favorite cakes, but without any added sugar. Full-fat Greek yogurt is one of my go-to ingredients, as it's full of vitamins and minerals (especially calcium) and protein, plus the probiotics are essential for a healthy gut.

1 Place all the ingredients in a blender and blend until smooth. For a lighter consistency, you can add a little more soy milk or water. Pour into your favorite glass and enjoy.

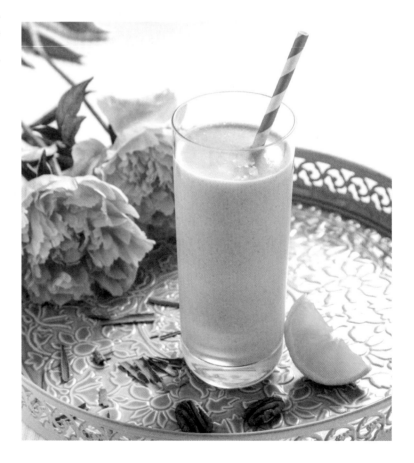

BANANA SPICED SMOOTHIE

2 tsp chia seeds

1 vanilla pod

3 tbsp full-fat Greek yogurt OR Greek-style soy-based vegan yogurt

scant 1 cup (200ml) unsweetened soy milk OR unsweetened pea milk

1 ripe banana, chopped

handful of ice cubes

FOR THE SPICE MIX

pinch of cinnamon

pinch of allspice

pinch of ground ginger

pinch of ground cloves

pinch of ground cardamom

This is just the thing to try if you want to spice up your regular smoothie habit with flavors of the Caribbean (and who wouldn't?). Bananas are high in potassium, which, along with many other benefits, helps muscles contract and regulate your heartbeat, as well as helping relieve anxiety and stress.

1 First, make the spice mix. Place all the spices in a bowl and mix together thoroughly.

2 Add half the chia seeds to the bowl, then slice the vanilla pod in half with a sharp knife and scrape the seeds in. Mix together thoroughly.

3 Place the yogurt, soy/pea milk, and banana in a blender and blend until smooth. Add the spice mix along with a handful of ice cubes and blend again.

4 Pour the smoothie into your favorite tall glass or travel mug and enjoy!

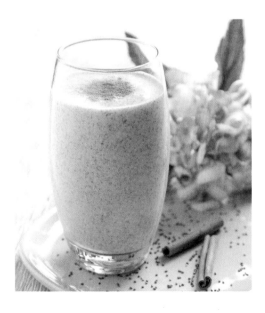

QUINOLA

SERVES TWO

2½oz (80g) quinoa (9oz/250g cooked weight)

1 tbsp chia seeds

1 tbsp mixed seeds (e.g., sunflowers seeds, flax seeds, poppy seeds: you can buy them premixed at most supermarkets)

1 heaping tsp dried blueberries

1 heaping tsp dried cranberries

12 almonds, roughly chopped

1 generous tsp honey

3 tbsp full-fat Greek yogurt OR Greek-style soy-based vegan yogurt OR 1 scant cup (200ml) unsweetened soy milk OR unsweetened pea milk (per serving)

When I started my health journey, I was amazed by the benefits of quinoa but wasn't sure how I could make the most of it as an ingredient. However, this recipe bakes it with nuts, seeds, and dried fruit so that you have a deliciously crunchy and healthy version of granola! Although it takes a little practice, this creation is one of my favorites, so make sure you give it a try!

1 Preheat the oven to 275°F and line a baking sheet with parchment paper.

2 Bring a pot of water to a boil and cook the quinoa according to the package instructions, about 20 minutes.

3 Place the cooked quinoa in a large bowl with all the seeds, dried fruit, and almonds and mix together well.

4 Stir in the honey, ensuring it coats every little bit of the mixture until it is all good and sticky.

5 Pour the mixture into the prepared tray and spread out evenly. Bake in the oven for 30 minutes, checking regularly and stirring every 10 minutes or so to ensure it is baking evenly. The mixture should be golden but not burned at all. (I like to turn the oven off and leave the quinola on the tray overnight for extra crunchiness.)

6 Remove from the oven and set aside to cool, then store in an airtight container until you are ready to serve.

7 Serve with Greek yogurt, soy milk, or pea milk.

GOOD TO KNOW

You can buy packages of precooked quinoa and use straight from the package. If you cook it at home, allow it to cool first to get that good crunch.

CHILI CHOCOLATE POWER PORRIDGE

SERVES ONE

½ serving (1 scoop/40ml) of The Six Pack Revolution Decadent Chocolate Caramel Post Workout Smoothie

1 scant cup (200ml) unsweetened almond milk

pinch of chili powder

4 heaping tbsp rolled oats

1 tsp natural peanut or almond butter (no added salt or sugar)

a few peanuts, chopped

This is a Six Pack Revolution favorite—delicious, filling, and a healthy way to satisfy chocolate cravings. Nut butters can be a great ingredient to have in the pantry; they're packed full of fiber and healthy fats. However, some brands can include palm oil, which is 50 percent saturated fat, so it is important to check the label.

1 Mix the protein shake, milk, and chili powder together and pour over the oats in a bowl. Cover and refrigerate overnight.

2 When you are ready to serve, warm in the microwave (if you like), top with your favorite nut butter and a sprinkling of peanuts, and enjoy!

GOOD TO KNOW

You need to prepare your oats the night before.

CHIA SEED SPECIAL

SERVES ONE

2 tbsp chia seeds

½ cup (125ml) unsweetened soy milk or unsweetened pea milk

1 tbsp full-fat Greek yogurt OR Greek-style soy-based vegan yogurt

1 tsp honey

1 vanilla bean, split and seeds removed

½ tsp ground cinnamon

½ handful of fresh mixed blueberries, raspberries, and/or blackberries

handful of mixed seeds of your choice

sprinkle of flaked, toasted almonds

sprig of fresh mint

Chia seeds are often described as little powerhouses of nutrition, as they're packed full of protein, fiber, omega-3 fats, and micronutrients. When you add honey, fresh berries, seeds, spices, and toasted nuts, you create a super-charged bowl of health! However, do plan ahead with this recipe, as the seeds need to soak for at least 3 hours, or overnight.

1 Slice the vanilla bean lengthwise and scrape out the vanilla bean seeds and paste. Set aside. (You can save the pod for infusing milk later.)

2 In a bowl, place the chia seeds, unsweetened soya milk, Greek yogurt, honey, vanilla paste, and cinnamon and mix together well. Cover and refrigerate for at least 3 hours, or overnight.

3 To serve, garnish with fresh berries and mixed seeds of your choice (I love pumpkin seeds for an extra crunch), almonds, and a sprig of fresh mint.

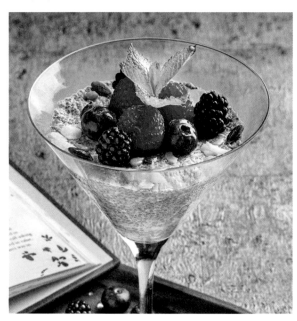

GOOD TO KNOW

I love to grow my own mint, just like my basil and other fresh herbs, as it always feels good to add homegrown herbs to my recipes!

CHOCOLATE AND HAZELNUT QUINOLA

2½oz (80g) quinoa (9oz/250g cooked weight)

1 tbsp chia seeds

1 tbsp cacao nibs

12 hazelnuts

½ serving (1 scoop/40ml) of The Six Pack Revolution Decadent Chocolate Caramel Post Workout Smoothie

1 heaping tsp honey

PER SERVING

3 tbsp full-fat Greek yogurt OR Greek-style soy-based vegan yogurt OR 1 scant cup (200ml) unsweetened soy/pea milk

Breakfast? Lunch? Bedtime snack? Any time is the perfect time for this little beauty. The cacao nibs make you feel like you're really indulging, yet they're exceptionally rich in antioxidants, so they deliver health benefits to boot.

1 Preheat the oven to 275°F and line a baking sheet with parchment paper.

2 Bring a pot of water to a boil and cook the quinoa according to the package instructions, about 20 minutes.

3 Place the cooked quinoa, chia seeds, cacao nibs, hazelnuts, and smoothie powder in a bowl and mix well.

4 Drizzle in the honey and mix together thoroughly.

5 Pour the mixture onto the prepared baking sheet and spread out evenly, then transfer to the oven and cook for 30 minutes, checking every 10 minutes to stir and respread the mixture each time.

6 Once the sticky mixture is golden brown, remove from the oven and set aside to cool completely. Alternatively, for an extra crunch, simply turn off the oven and leave the mixture to cool overnight.

7 Serve with your choice of yogurt or milk.

GOOD TO KNOW

You can buy packages of cooked quinoa that are ready-to-use.

RASPBERRY AND FIG MUESLI

8 tbsp rolled oats

8 tbsp barley flakes

2 tbsp chia seeds

2 tbsp mixed seeds

36 hazelnuts, chopped

handful of whole dried raspberries

3 soft dried figs, finely chopped

PER SERVING

3 tbsp full-fat Greek yogurt OR Greek-style soy-based vegan yogurt OR 1 scant cup (200ml) unsweetened soy/pea milk

Muesli is often thought of as being healthy, and yet many brands are so high in added sugar and salt that they really don't qualify. However, this version is full of delicious nuts and seeds, and the dried fruit provides all the sweetness that you need.

1 Preheat the oven to 275°F and line a baking sheet with parchment paper.

2 In a bowl, mix the oats, barley, chia seeds, and chopped hazelnuts together, then pour the mixture onto the prepared baking sheet and spread out evenly.

3 Bake in the oven for 10 minutes, then stir and respread the mixture before returning to the oven for another 8 minutes. Remove from the oven and set aside to cool completely.

4 Once cooled, mix in the dried fruit and serve with your choice of yogurt, soy milk, or pea milk.

5 This recipe makes a big batch. Stored in an airtight container, it should keep for up to 3 weeks.

GOOD TO KNOW

You can often buy bags of premixed seeds at most supermarkets. Look for ones that include sunflower, flax, poppy, pumpkin, or hemp seeds.

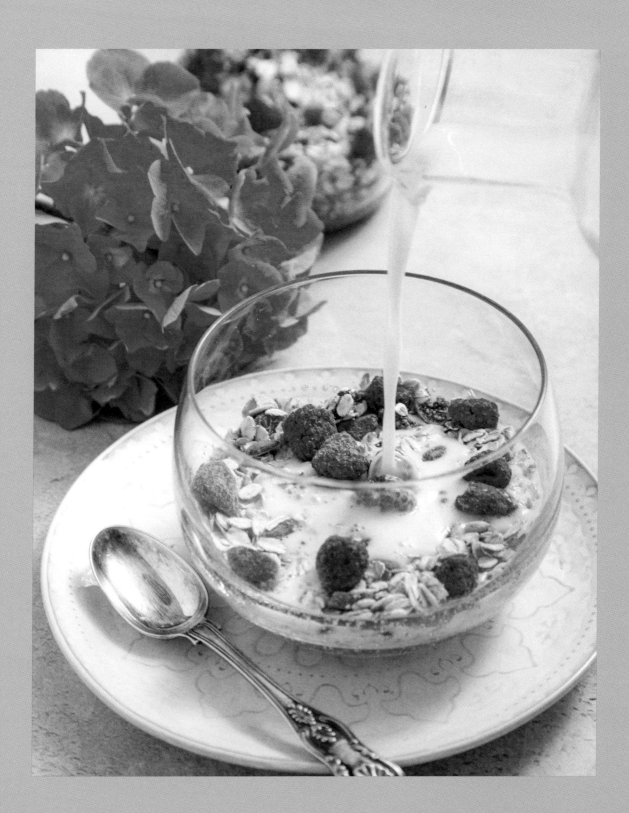

PEACHY PORRIDGE

SERVES FOUR

FOR THE PORRIDGE MIX

2½oz (75g) dry quinoa

11½oz (45g) rolled oats

3 tbsp flaked, toasted almonds

4 cardamom pods

PER SERVING

1 scant cup (200ml) unsweetened soy or pea milk

1 ripe peach, cut into wedges

1 tbsp full-fat Greek yogurt OR plain sugar-free yogurt OR Greek-style soy-based vegan yogurt

zest of 1 orange, plus a squeeze of juice

I love how fragrant this porridge is, with almonds and cardamom, and the delicate fruitiness of the grilled peach tops it to perfection. In fact, this recipe perfectly illustrates one of my main maxims—that no meal should be naked!—as spices add not only flavor but also health benefits. Cardamom is a great spice, as it pairs so well with fruit, but is also high in magnesium and zinc and great at fighting inflammation. Peaches are also full of vitamins A and C, and I recommend you keep the skin on, for maximum fiber.

1 First, make up your porridge mix. In a bowl, combine the dry quinoa, rolled oats, and almonds and mix. Smash the cardamom pods and add the seeds and pods to the mix, stirring again to distribute evenly.

2 For each serving, spoon 3 tablespoons of porridge mix into a small saucepan. Add 1 scant cup (200ml) soy or pea milk and gently bring to a boil, then reduce the heat and simmer until you have the consistency that you like.

3 While the porridge is simmering, place the peach slices cut-side down onto a hot ridged grill pan and cook until lightly caramelized (turning frequently).

4 Remove the cardamom pods (not great to crunch on) from your porridge and serve topped with peach slices, a dollop of Greek yogurt, a sprinkle of orange zest, and a squeeze of orange juice.

GOOD TO KNOW

The dry porridge mix can be stored in an airtight container for up to 2 weeks.

POWER PORRIDGE

SERVES ONE

½ serving (1 scoop/40ml) of The
Six Pack Revolution Vanilla
Caramel Heaven Post Workout
Smoothie

a generous ½ cup (150ml)
unsweetened almond milk
OR water

¼ tsp ground cinnamon

4 tbsp rolled oats

1 tsp natural cashew butter OR
any natural nut butter

pinch of ground cinnamon

This power porridge contains the perfect balance of protein and healthy carbohydrates to help you feel full of energy. It's a great way to start your day, or for any other time when you feel your energy levels need an extra, sustainable boost.

1 Place the post workout smoothie, almond milk, and cinnamon in a blender and blend until smooth. Place the oats in a bowl, pour in the blended mix, and stir, then cover and refrigerate overnight.

2 Serve with a spoonful of nut butter and a sprinkle of cinnamon.

GOOD TO KNOW

This recipe ideally needs to be refrigerated overnight, so ensure you plan ahead.

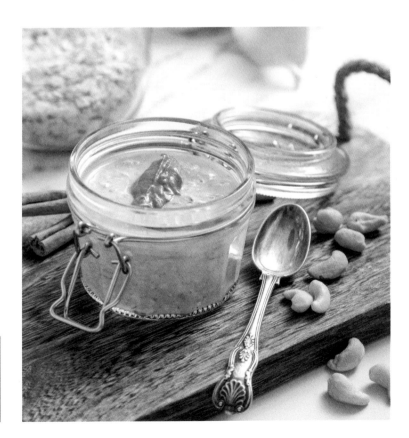

OATOLA

SERVES TWO

6 tbsp jumbo rolled oats

1 tbsp flax seeds

1 tbsp chia seeds

12 unsalted pecan halves

1 heaping tsp honey

handful of freeze-dried apple

¼ tsp cinnamon

PER SERVING

3 tbsp full-fat Greek yogurt OR Greek-style soy-based vegan yogurt OR 1 scant cup (200ml) unsweetened soy/pea milk

Granola is another breakfast staple, like muesli, that can be corrupted by excess added sugar. Therefore, I always prefer to make my own, with lots of healthy nuts and seeds and minimal sweetness. In fact, freeze-dried fruits add a lovely natural sweet flavor. They contain 97 percent of the nutrients of fresh fruit and are healthier than dried fruits, which can lose more nutrients through heat treatment.

1 Preheat the oven to 275°F and line a baking sheet with parchment paper.

2 In a bowl, mix the oats, seeds, and pecans together, then drizzle in the honey and stir until everything is thoroughly coated. Pour the mixture onto the prepared tray and spread out evenly.

3 Bake in the oven for 10 minutes, then stir and respread the mixture before returning to the oven for another 8 minutes. Remove from the oven and set aside to cool completely.

4 Once cooled, mix in the freeze-dried apple and cinnamon and serve with your choice of yogurt, soy milk, or pea milk.

GOOD TO KNOW

Stored in an airtight container in the fridge, your granola will keep for up to 2 weeks. Don't leave at room temperature, as the nuts release their natural oils and the mixture can get a little "greasy."

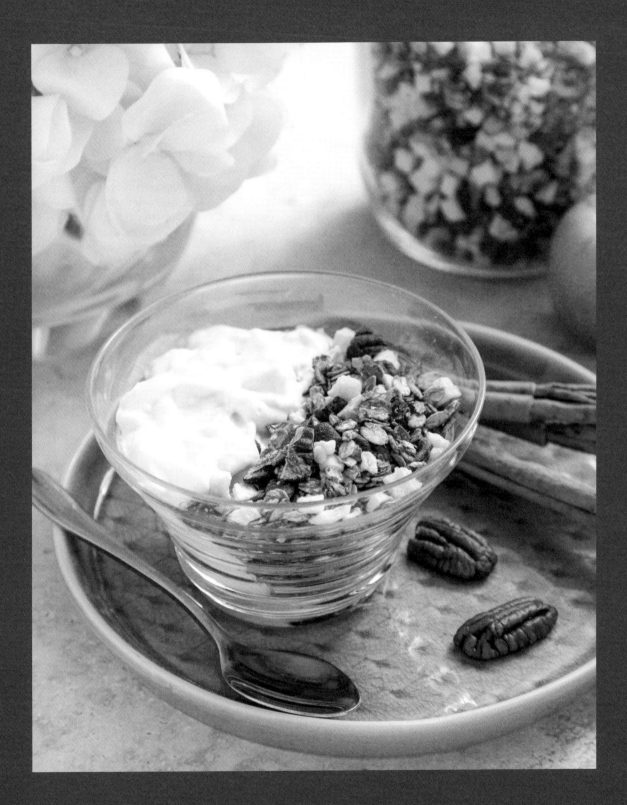

YOGURT
AND BERRIES

SERVES ONE

3 tbsp full-fat Greek yogurt
OR Greek-style soy-based
vegan yogurt

handful of blueberries,
blackberries, OR raspberries
(or a mix of all three)

6 almonds

sprig of fresh mint, to garnish

This makes the simplest and tastiest snack but is so full of goodness. I always keep lots of berries in the freezer, as many studies have proven that they contain as much nutrition as freshly picked berries, and you can eat them all year-round.

1 Spoon the yogurt into your favorite dish and sprinkle the berries and almonds over the top. Garnish with a sprig of mint and enjoy.

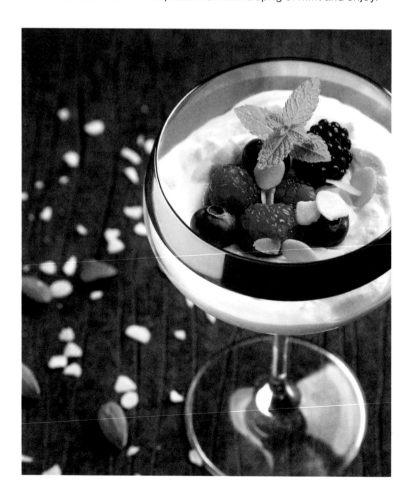

TROPICAL FRUIT SALAD

SERVES ONE

combined handful of chopped
pineapple, kiwi, and passion
fruit

3 tbsp full-fat Greek yogurt
OR Greek-style soy-based
vegan yogurt

2 tsp coconut shavings or dried,
shredded coconut

Oh boy, this is simple but also the tastiest way to deliver a major vitamin C boost with lots of health-promoting antioxidants!

1 Place a spoonful of yogurt in a glass or bowl, then layer with some fruit and then coconut, and keep on layering until the ingredients are used up. This way, you get a little bit of deliciousness with every spoonful! Serve right away.

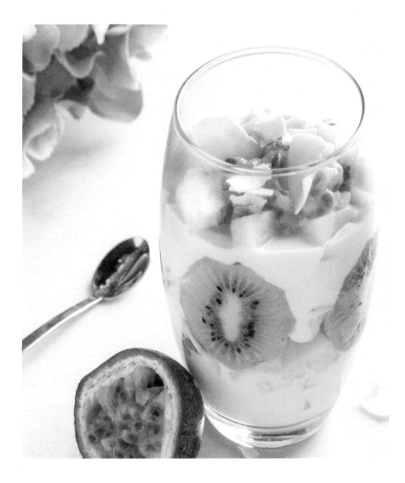

WONDERFUL WAFFLES

SERVES ONE

2 eggs, beaten

1 tbsp full-fat cottage cheese

2 tbsp rolled oats

6½ tbsp (100ml) soy milk

1 tsp chia seeds

1 banana (½ mashed and ½ sliced)

1 tsp coconut oil, for oiling

1 tbsp full-fat Greek yogurt OR Greek-style soy-based vegan yogurt

zest and juice of ½ lemon

pinch of ground cinnamon

Waffles aren't generally the healthiest option for breakfast, as they're traditionally made with refined white flour, butter, and lots of sugar. However, these are made with rolled oats and cottage cheese instead, which is what makes them wonderful. Cottage cheese is an essential ingredient for me, as it's full of protein and calcium, yet contains relatively few calories.

1 Preheat a waffle maker.

2 Place the beaten eggs in a blender with the cottage cheese, oats, soy milk, and chia seeds, then puree until you have a smooth batter.

3 Add the mashed banana and blend briefly again.

4 Lightly oil the waffle maker, then pour in the mixture and cook for approximately 5–6 minutes, until ready.

5 Serve each waffle with sliced banana, a spoonful of Greek yogurt, and a squeeze of lemon juice. Sprinkle the lemon zest and cinnamon over the top.

GOOD TO KNOW

You can use this recipe to make pancakes—cook in a non-stick skillet for 2–3 minutes on each side.

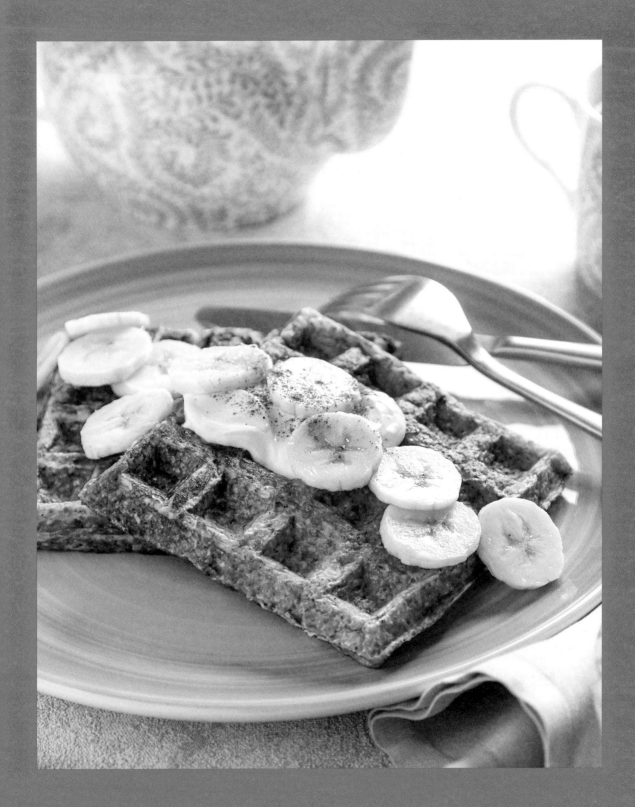

ORANGE AND LEMON POPPY SEED PANCAKES

3 egg whites

1 vanilla bean

3 tbsp oats, blended into a powder

zest and juice of ½ lemon, plus 4 thin slices to garnish

zest and juice of ½ orange, plus 4 thin slices to garnish

1 tbsp poppy seeds

2 tbsp full-fat cottage cheese

1 tsp coconut oil

1 tbsp full-fat Greek yogurt OR Greek-style soy-based vegan yogurt

8 pistachios, crushed or chopped

With these pancakes, the sweetness of the orange balances the sourness of the lemon, so there is no need for sugar. I also like to use oats instead of refined white flour, as it contains more fiber, protein, and nutrients. It's so easy to make at home, plus oats are digested slowly, so they keep you feeling full.

1 Slice the vanilla bean lengthwise and scrape out the vanilla bean seeds and paste. Set aside. (You can save the pod for infusing milk later.)

2 In a large bowl, blend the egg whites with the vanilla bean paste until frothy. Add the oats, lemon and orange zest, and juice along with the poppy seeds and blend again. Finally, fold the cottage cheese into the batter mix until thoroughly incorporated.

3 Heat a little coconut oil in a non-stick skillet over medium heat. When hot, add a ladleful of batter and swirl the pan until the base is evenly coated. Cook the pancake for 2–3 minutes, then flip over and cook the other side until golden brown.

4 Serve each pancake with a heaping teaspoon of Greek yogurt and a sprinkle of pistachios on top. Garnish with slices of orange and lemon.

RASPBERRY AND BLUEBERRY PANCAKES

SERVES ONE

4 egg whites

1 vanilla bean

large pinch of ground cinnamon

3 tbsp oats

large handful of blueberries

2 tbsp full-fat cottage cheese

large handful of raspberries

1 tsp coconut oil

All types of berries are a superfood, as they are full of vitamins —especially vitamin C, which boosts your immune system— plus antioxidants called flavonoids, which fight inflammation. These simple pancakes include both blueberries and raspberries and make a perfect healthy snack.

1 Slice the vanilla bean lengthwise and scrape out the vanilla bean seeds and paste. Set aside. (You can save the pod for infusing milk later.)

2 In a large bowl, blend the egg whites with the vanilla bean paste and cinnamon until frothy. Add the oats and blueberries and blend again. Finally, fold the cottage cheese into the batter mix until thoroughly incorporated.

3 Place 5 raspberries in a bowl and mash with a fork until you have a bright, glossy pulp, then set aside.

4 Heat a little coconut oil in a non-stick skillet over medium heat. When hot, add a ladleful of batter and swirl the pan until the base is evenly coated. Cook the pancake for 2–3 minutes, then flip over and cook the other side until golden brown.

5 Serve each pancake with a drizzle of raspberry jus and a scattering of fresh raspberries.

HOT BREAKFAST WITH SWEET POTATO HASH BROWNS

SERVES ONE

2–3 eggs

handful of thickly grated sweet potato

handful of fresh spinach

½ avocado, sliced

freshly ground black pepper

A large hot breakfast with hash browns isn't always the healthiest choice on a breakfast menu, but with this recipe that's full of protein, iron-rich spinach, and healthy fats, I've made sure it is. Sweet potato is incredibly rich in vitamin A, plus it contains more fiber than a white potato, so it keeps you full for longer and doesn't result in such a sharp blood sugar spike. Serve with poached eggs, or if you fancy something different, try frying them in water (see Tip below).

1 First, make the hash browns. Beat one egg in a bowl and mix in the grated sweet potato, then use your hands to shape into two small patties.

2 Heat a non-stick skillet over moderate heat and fry the hash browns for approximately 8–10 minutes, until golden brown and crispy on both sides.

3 Now, poach the eggs. Bring a pan of water to a boil, then reduce the heat until it is barely simmering. Crack one egg into a cup and slide it gently into the water, then repeat with the final remaining egg. Cook for 2–3 minutes, then lift each egg out of the water with a slotted spoon and drain them on kitchen paper.

4 Now, wilt your spinach. I like to wilt my spinach for a few minutes in a dry saucepan—no water in sight. It keeps the spinach from getting watery and holds in all that iron-rich flavor.

5 Arrange the hash browns on a serving dish and top with the poached eggs. Add the avocado and wilted spinach and season with black pepper.

GOOD TO KNOW

I like my eggs poached and slightly runny, but you can also hard-boil them, scramble them, or fry them in water. To fry, simply cover the base of a frying pan with boiling water instead of oil.

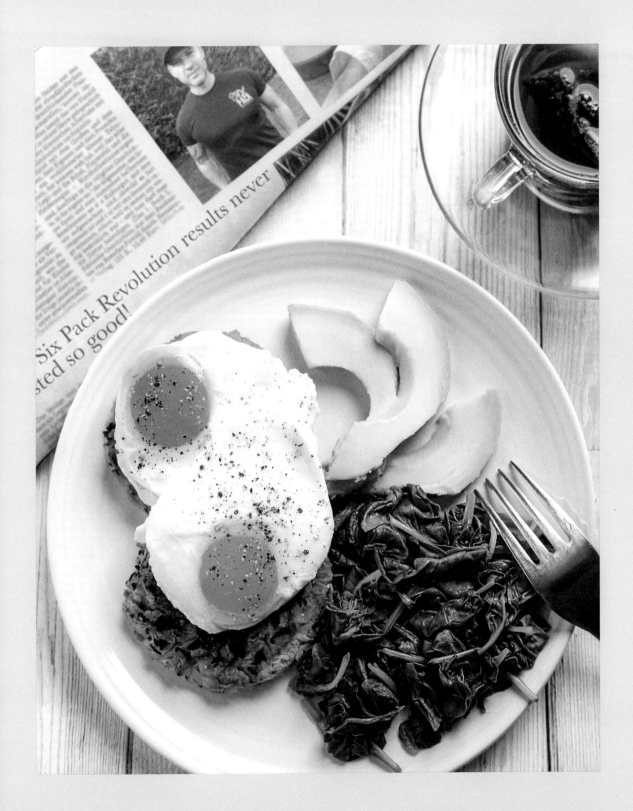

SCRAMBLED EGGS, SPINACH AND AVOCADO

2–3 eggs

handful of spinach

½ avocado, sliced

freshly ground black pepper

Eggs are considered a perfect protein source, and scrambling them is the one thing you just can't get wrong. This simple dish contains the perfect balance of protein, carbs, and healthy fats that will keep you feeling full and nourished—and also help muscles to grow and repair.

1 Whisk the eggs together in a small bowl.

2 Pour the beaten egg into a non-stick skillet over medium heat and cook, stirring constantly, until it has almost reached your preferred consistency. At this point, add the spinach and continue to stir, then take the pan off the heat.

3 Serve the scrambled eggs with sliced avocado, season with black pepper, and enjoy!

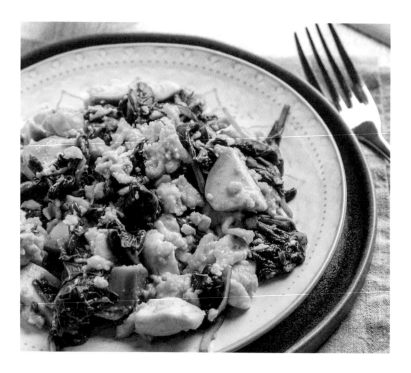

BOILED EGGS
AND **SOLDIERS**

SERVES ONE

2–3 eggs

1 tsp extra virgin olive oil

handful of asparagus spears

freshly ground black pepper

I love to eat this simple breakfast on a Sunday morning while reading the weekend paper and generally indulging in some family time! Eggs are, of course, an excellent source of protein, and the asparagus is not only packed with free-radical fighting antioxidants but also low in calories and beneficial for those who need to keep an eye on blood sugar levels/blood pressure.

1 Bring a pan of water to a boil and cook the eggs for approximately 6–8 minutes, depending on how you like them. If you like a runny yolk and wobbly white, 6 minutes should do it. A minute longer will set the white, and by 8 minutes, the yolk will start to set too.

2 Meanwhile, place a non-stick skillet or ridged grill pan over medium-high heat. Toss the asparagus spears in the oil, then lay them in the pan and cook, turning frequently, until they soften and char slightly.

3 Using a small spoon, slice the top off the eggs, season with some black pepper, and dunk away!

GOOD TO KNOW

It's important not to overcook the asparagus for two reasons: It will lose many essential nutrients and become floppy, and therefore be useless as soldiers for your eggs!

SHAKSHUKA

SERVES ONE

1 tsp extra virgin olive oil

½ small red onion, chopped

1 garlic clove, crushed

½ red pepper, chopped

½ portobello mushroom cap, sliced

½ tsp mild chili powder

pinch of cayenne pepper

pinch of paprika

½ tsp ground cumin

7oz/200g chopped tomatoes (½ x 14oz/411g can)

2–3 eggs

freshly ground black pepper

1 heaping tsp fresh, finely chopped cilantro

Shakshuka is a classic Middle Eastern dish, and its name literally means "all mixed up." It is cooked in one pot and can be eaten at any time of the day, as it works just as well for brunch as for dinner. I love its ultra-fragrant and warming flavors and the fact that it is all so healthy!

1 Heat the oil in a non-stick skillet that has a lid over moderate heat and fry the onion, garlic, pepper, and mushroom until soft and the onion starts to caramelize.

2 Stir in the spices and cook for a minute until fragrant, then add the chopped tomatoes and bring to a simmer. Cook for approximately 3 minutes.

3 Using a wooden spoon, make three wells in the sauce and then crack an egg into each one. Cover the pan with a lid and cook for 8–10 minutes, until the eggs are done to your liking.

4 Season with black pepper and scatter fresh cilantro over the top. I like to eat it straight from the pan, but you can also transfer to a nice bowl!

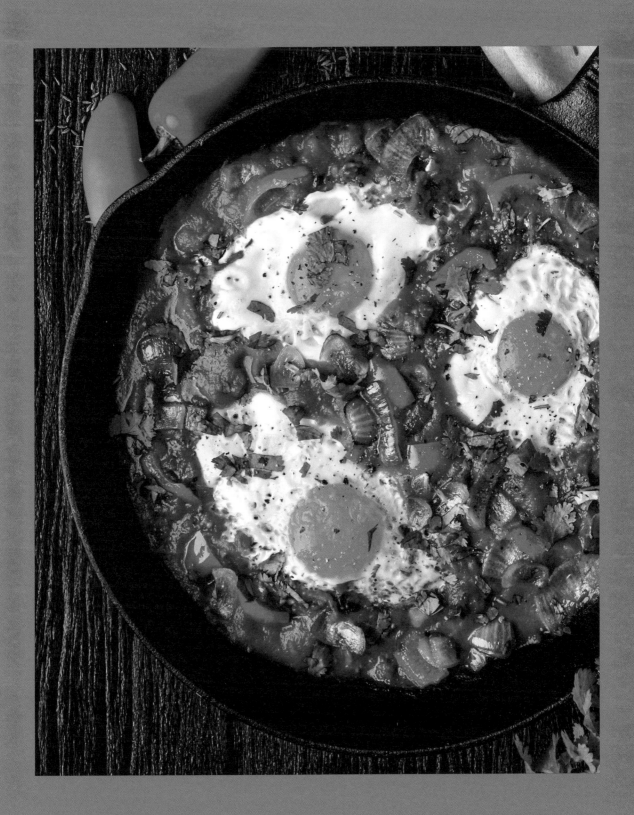

FULLY LOADED FRITTATA

SERVES THREE

3 tsp extra virgin olive oil

6–9 eggs

½ tsp Italian seasoning

small handful of chopped broccoli

small handful of sliced zucchini

1 red pepper, thinly sliced

1 red onion, chopped

handful of fresh spinach

pinch of chili flakes (optional)

Frittatas are great when you're looking for a powerful hit of energy and healthy nutrients—I've loaded this one with superfoods like broccoli and spinach. They're also super-easy to put together, and I even love to eat them cold, so do swap your sandwich habit for a slice of tasty frittata—it's the perfect grab-and-go lunch.

1 Preheat the oven to 350°F and grease a wide, shallow ovenproof dish with 1 teaspoon of oil.

2 Crack the eggs into a large bowl and whisk together with the Italian seasoning. Add all the vegetables with the remaining extra virgin olive oil and mix well.

3 Transfer the mixture to your ovenproof dish and bake in the oven for 30–40 minutes, until the frittata is cooked through and starting to brown on the top.

4 Allow the frittata to cool slightly in the pan before you transfer to a plate, slice, and serve.

GOOD TO KNOW

Add some chili flakes if you'd like a little heat kick! Store any leftovers in the fridge in a sealed container for 2–3 days.

SPINACH AND ASPARAGUS OMELET

SERVES ONE

1 tsp extra virgin olive oil

3 asparagus spears, sliced in half lengthwise

2–3 eggs, beaten

freshly ground black pepper

small handful of fresh baby spinach

1 heaping tsp fresh, finely chopped cilantro

Omelets are awesome and my favorite kind of fast food. They take just minutes to prepare, are so full of protein that you stay feeling full, plus they're incredibly versatile—you can add all types of tasty vegetables, cheeses, and herbs, so you need never get bored.

1 Heat the oil in a non-stick pan over moderate heat and fry the asparagus spears until they have lightly charred.

2 In a bowl, beat the eggs with a fork and season with black pepper. Arrange the asparagus in the pan so it is evenly spaced, then pour the egg mixture on top and tilt the pan slightly so the eggs cover the surface of the pan completely. With a spatula, push the edges toward the center of the pan and keep tilting the pan so the runny egg moves to the edges and cooks through.

3 When the omelette mixture is set to your liking, run the spatula around the edge of the pan to help free the omelette, then slide it onto a serving plate.

4 Cover half of the omelet with the spinach, then fold over. Season with more black pepper and a sprinkling of cilantro and enjoy immediately.

BOMBAY POTATO OMELET

SERVES ONE

½ sweet potato (skin on), diced

1 tsp extra virgin olive oil

½ small red onion OR 1 shallot, chopped

1 tsp curry powder

1 tsp chia seeds, plus extra to garnish

pinch of white pepper

3 cherry tomatoes, quartered

handful of spinach leaves

2–3 eggs

splash of unsweetened soy milk OR unsweetened pea milk

wedge of lemon

salt and freshly ground white pepper

fresh, finely chopped cilantro, to garnish

FOR THE RAITA

14oz (400g) full-fat Greek yogurt OR Greek-style soy-based vegan yogurt

½ cucumber, grated and lightly squeezed to remove excess water

½ bunch fresh cilantro, finely chopped

½ bunch fresh mint, finely chopped

½ tsp garam masala

1–2 garlic cloves, crushed

½ lime, squeezed

GOOD TO KNOW

The raita recipe will make more than is needed, but you can store or freeze the rest for another meal. Stored in an airtight container, it will keep in the fridge for a few days, or in the freezer for up to a month.

This filling and flavorsome recipe is one of our most popular, as it just keeps on giving. The curry flavor works so well with the eggs and potatoes, and the accompaniment of the herb-filled and creamy raita provides such a contrast that all tastebuds are satisfied!

1 Bring a pot of water to a boil and cook the sweet potato for around 8 minutes, until soft, then drain and set aside.

2 Heat the oil in a non-stick saute pan over low heat and cook the onion until it caramelizes—this slow cooking will allow it to release all its delicious sweetness.

3 While the onion is caramelizing, make the raita. Simply place all the ingredients in a bowl and stir to combine thoroughly.

4 Add sweet potatoes to the onion mixture and saute until it browns, then stir in the curry powder, chia seeds, white pepper, cherry tomatoes, and half of the spinach leaves along with a splash of water, then stir all the ingredients for a couple of minutes.

5 Once the spinach has wilted a little, take the pan off the heat and transfer the mixture to a bowl. Cover and keep warm.

6 Crack the eggs into a separate bowl and beat well with a fork. Add a splash of soy or pea milk, stir, and then pour the mixture into the original saute pan, tilting it slightly so that the eggs cover the surface of the pan completely. With a spatula, push the edges toward the center of the pan and keep tilting the pan so the runny egg moves to the edges and cooks through.

7 When the omelet begins to set, spread the prepared filling over one side, then fold the other side over the top.

8 Place the remaining spinach on a serving plate and, when the omelet is cooked, run the spatula around the edge of the pan and slide it on top of the bed of spinach. Serve with a lemon wedge and a spoonful of raita and garnish with fresh cilantro and a pinch of chia seeds, if you wish.

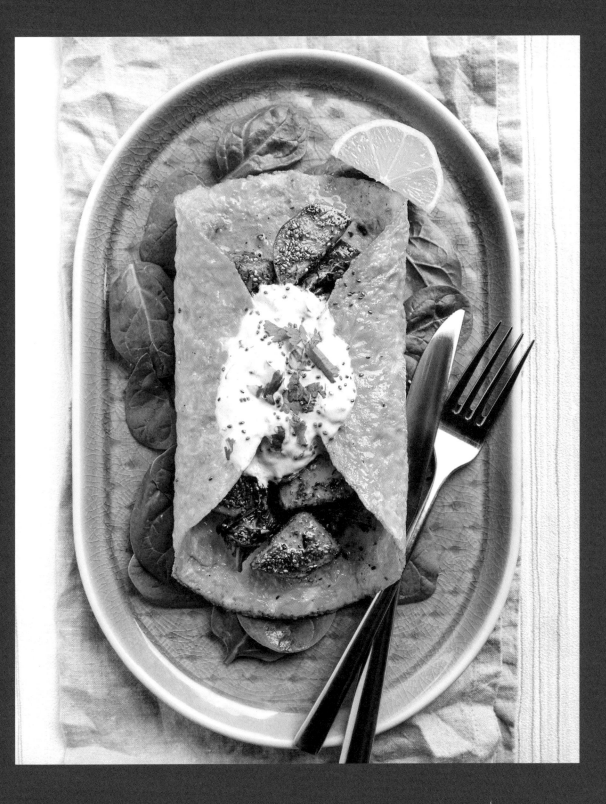

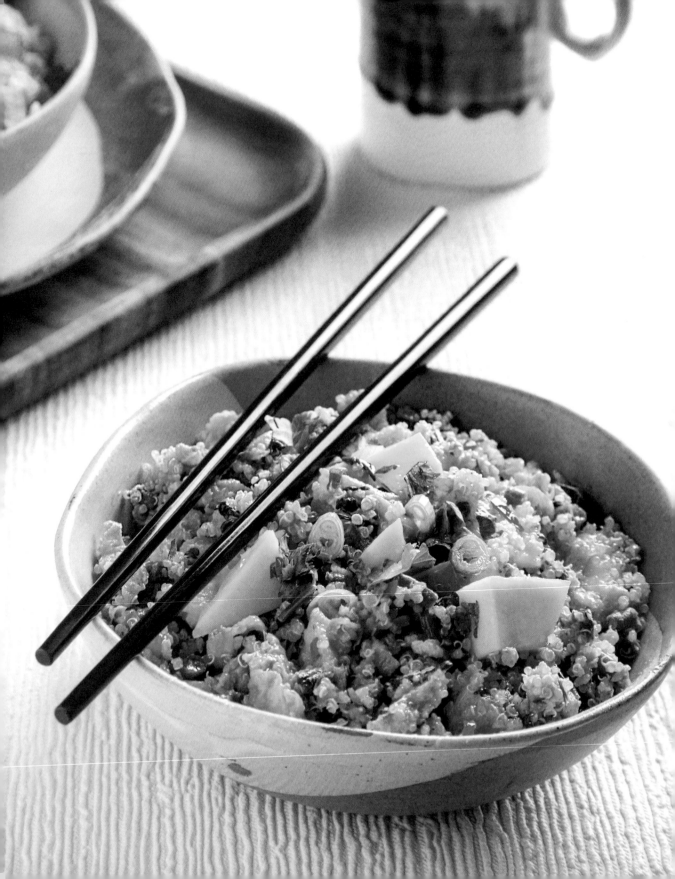

EGG FRIED NICE

2oz (60g) quinoa (180g ready cooked weight)

1 tsp sesame oil

2 garlic cloves, crushed

2 green onions, sliced

small handful of green beans, chopped

1 tbsp fresh, finely chopped cilantro, plus a little extra to garnish

4 cherry tomatoes, quartered

½ small zucchini, chopped

1 fresh chili, deseeded and finely chopped

1 tsp grated fresh ginger root

pinch of white pepper

1 tsp extra virgin olive oil

4–6 eggs, beaten

½ small mango, chopped into small pieces

A Chinese takeout egg-fried rice isn't all that authentic or healthy, as it's often cooked with lots of oil and salt. However, it doesn't have to be that way, and this recipe shows how you can make it with nutrient-dense whole grains and pack it with veggies for an incredibly satisfying takeout-style classic.

1 First, bring a pot of water to a boil and cook the quinoa according to the package instructions, about 20 minutes. Set aside.

2 Heat the sesame oil in a non-stick skillet over medium heat and add the garlic, green onions, green beans, cilantro, tomatoes, zucchini, chili, ginger, and white pepper. Cook, stirring, until the ingredients soften, then add the cooked quinoa and stir to combine. Transfer the mixture to a bowl and set aside.

3 Now, make the omelet. Heat the olive oil in the same skillet over medium heat and add the beaten eggs, tilting the pan slightly so that the eggs cover the surface completely. With a spatula, push the edges toward the center of the pan and keep tilting the pan so the runny egg moves to the edges and cooks through.

4 When the omelet is cooked through, slide it onto a plate and chop into small pieces.

5 Return all the ingredients to the skillet, together with the chopped mango, and toss everything together over low heat to gently warm through.

6 Serve in your favorite bowl and garnish with fresh cilantro.

BOMBAY MIX

SERVES TWO

15.5oz (439g) can of chickpeas, drained and rinsed

½ tsp cumin seeds

½ tsp fennel seeds

½ tsp mustard seeds

2 tsp unsalted peanuts

handful of raisins

1 tsp pine nuts

1 tsp curry leaves

1 tsp curry powder

1 tsp garam masala

½ tsp chili powder

These roasted, slightly crunchy, spice-coated chickpeas are the perfect healthy version of Indian Bombay mix and ideal for snacking at any time of day. Many studies have shown that the sensory pleasures we experience from the taste of food can be a big factor in determining how much we eat, which is why I love spices so much—they're guaranteed to satisfy our tastebuds and provide a sense of satiety.

1 Preheat the oven to 325°F and line a baking sheet with parchment paper.

2 Pat dry the chickpeas with paper towels to remove all excess moisture, then place in a bowl with the cumin, fennel, and mustard seeds and toss to ensure the chickpeas are thoroughly coated.

3 Transfer the chickpeas to the prepared baking sheet and spread out evenly.

4 Bake in the oven for 25–30 minutes, then remove and add all the remaining ingredients. Stir to mix well before returning the tray to the oven. Cook for another 10–15 minutes, then set aside to cool.

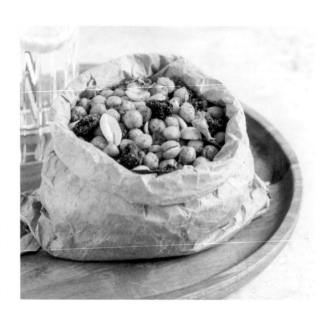

GOOD TO KNOW

Your mix can be stored in an airtight container until ready to eat and can be stored for up to a week!

HUMMUS
WITH CRUDITÉS

SERVES TWO

handful of crudités of your choice—we love red or yellow bell peppers, cucumber, and celery

pinch of paprika, to garnish (optional)

sprig of fresh cilantro, to garnish (optional)

FOR THE HUMMUS

15.5oz (439g) can of chickpeas, drained and rinsed

1 garlic clove, crushed

1 tsp extra virgin olive oil

juice of ½ lemon

½ tsp ground cumin

Hummus makes an excellent snack, both fiber-rich and full of plant-based protein. I always keep a container in the fridge and like to play around with the veggies that I make into crudités, using whatever is fresh and in season.

1 Place the chickpeas, garlic, olive oil, lemon juice, and cumin in a food processor and blend until you have the consistency you prefer. Add a tiny splash of water if you want to loosen it a little.

2 Serve with a handful of raw seasonal crudités of your choice and garnish with a good pinch of paprika and a sprig of cilantro.

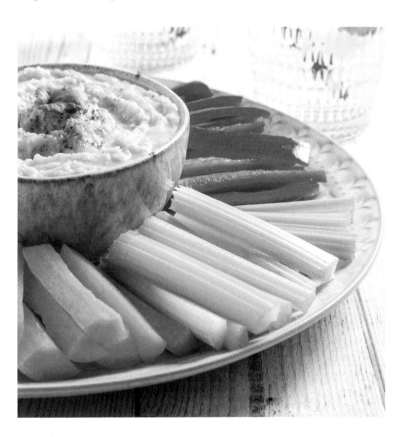

COTTAGE CHEESE
ON **RICE CAKES**

SERVES ONE

½ avocado, thinly sliced

2 rice cakes

3 tbsp full-fat cottage cheese

pomegranate seeds, to garnish

chopped chives, to garnish

This snack is as pretty as a picture and packed full of nutrients. The green goodness that is avocado contains more potassium than a banana, and the pomegranate seeds are stuffed full of antioxidants.

1 Lay the avocado slices on top of the rice cakes and spoon the cottage cheese on top. Sprinkle the pomegranate seeds and some chopped chives over the top—delicious!

GOOD TO KNOW

The remaining avocado half can be stored in the fridge for another day, either covered in plastic wrap or in an airtight container. Always leave the pit in to protect the flesh underneath.

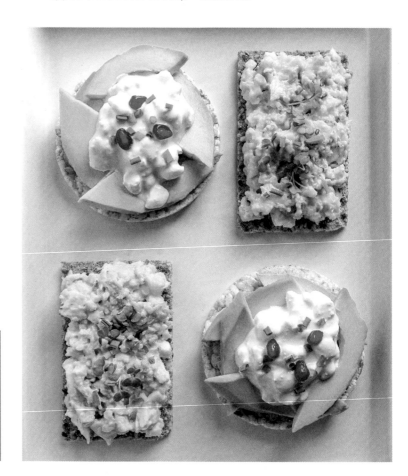

EGG AVONNAISE ON RYE CRISPBREAD

SERVES ONE

2–3 eggs

½ avocado

1 tbsp full-fat Greek yogurt OR Greek-style soy-based vegan yogurt

squeeze of lemon juice

1 tsp fresh chopped chives, plus a little more to garnish

pinch of fresh microgreens

2 rye crispbreads

freshly ground black pepper

Eggs are fantastic, as they're rich in protein and contain all 9 essential amino acids, yet mixing them with store-bought mayonnaise can downgrade the overall nutritional value of your meal. Therefore, this recipe replaces the mayo with avocado and Greek yogurt, which, in my opinion, is a masterstroke! With this substitution, you get all the creaminess of mayo, yet with heart-healthy unsaturated fats instead of saturated. I guarantee you won't miss the mayonnaise one bit.

1 First, boil the eggs. Bring a pot of water to a boil and cook the eggs for about 12 minutes—you want them to be hard so you can mash them. After 12 minutes, immediately transfer the eggs to a bowl of cold water to stop the cooking.

2 In a bowl, mash the avocado and combine with the Greek yogurt, lemon juice, and chopped chives.

3 When the eggs are cool enough to handle, peel the shells and mash the eggs, then add them to the bowl with the avocado and combine.

4 Spoon the mixture onto the crispbreads, sprinkle with some fresh microgreens, and season with black pepper. You will find that this makes a lot of egg avonnaise, so be sure to finish it all. Enjoy!

THAI FRUIT SKEWERS

SERVES TWO

$^2/_3$ cup (150ml) coconut milk

zest and juice of 1 lime

pinch of cayenne pepper

kiwi, pineapple, and mango, cut into cubes (approx. 2 handfuls)

1 tbsp fresh, finely chopped mint

4 tsp coconut flakes

PER SERVING

3 tbsp full-fat Greek yogurt OR Greek-style soy-based vegan yogurt

Infused with Thai flavors and as colorful as a glowing sun—simple fruit skewers have never looked or tasted so good!

1 Place the coconut milk, lime zest and juice, and cayenne pepper in a bowl. Add the fruit, ensuring it is all submerged, then transfer to the fridge and leave to infuse, stirring occasionally, for at least an hour.

2 Drain the marinade (this can be discarded) and thread the fruit onto two large skewers.

3 Sprinkle with fresh mint and coconut flakes and serve with yogurt for dipping!

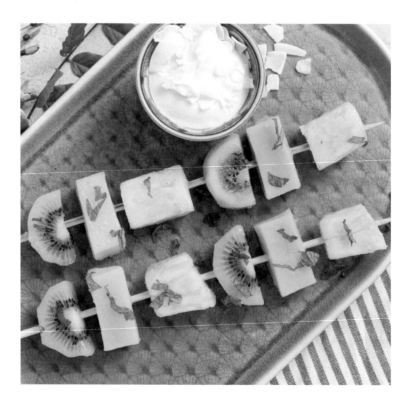

MIXED BERRY CRUMBLE

SERVES TWO

handful of blueberries (fresh or frozen)

3 tbsp rolled oats

½ serving (1 scoop; 40ml) of The Six Pack Revolution Vanilla Caramel Heaven Post Workout Smoothie

6 almonds, chopped

juice of 1 lemon

cinnamon (optional)

3 tbsp Greek yogurt OR Greek-style soy-based vegan yogurt, to serve

The Six Pack Revolution Vanilla Caramel Heaven Post Workout Smoothie brings both protein and flavor and, with cooked blueberries and a crunchy golden topping, makes this an outstanding and guilt-free dessert.

1 Preheat the oven to 350°F.

2 Place the blueberries in a small ovenproof ramekin-type dish so that they cover the bottom.

3 In a bowl, place the oats, smoothie powder, almonds, and lemon juice and, using your fingers, rub the ingredients together to create that crumble effect (it will be dry and sticky).

4 Spread the crumble mixture evenly over the fruit base and sprinkle with a little cinnamon (if using).

5 Transfer to the oven and bake for approximately 20 minutes, until the top has turned golden brown. Serve with a little Greek yogurt.

GOOD TO KNOW

For an extra crunchy and golden crumble top, place the dish under the broiler for another few minutes, but keep an eye on it, as it can burn very quickly.

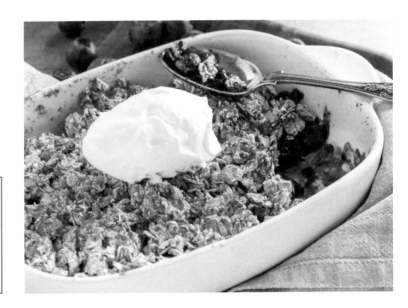

BANOOKIES

SERVES ONE

handful of chopped banana

½ serving (1 scoop; 40ml) of The Six Pack Revolution Decadent Chocolate Caramel Post Workout Smoothie

6 hazelnuts, chopped

What are banookies? Cookies with a difference, that's what! These are packed full of healthy protein and are delicious served warm or cold. This recipe makes four regular-sized cookies and they'll keep for a couple of days in an airtight container, if you don't eat them first!

1 Preheat the oven to 350°F and line a baking sheet with parchment paper.

2 Place the banana in a bowl and mash thoroughly with the back of a fork until you have a wet consistency. Mix in the smoothie powder and chopped hazelnuts to form a thick batter.

3 Using a spoon, drop cookie-sized amounts of the batter onto the prepared baking sheet, evenly spaced apart, and bake for 15–20 minutes. Check regularly to make sure they don't burn.

4 Remove from the oven and leave to cool on the tray for at least 10 minutes, then transfer to a cooling rack.

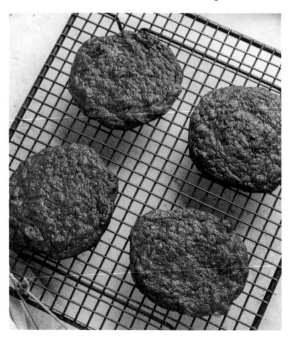

GRILLED NECTARINES

SERVES ONE

1 large nectarine, cut into 8 segments

3 tbsp full-fat Greek yogurt OR Greek-style soy-based vegan yogurt

zest and juice of ½ orange

8 pistachio nuts, chopped

You must try this even if you are not a fan of nectarines. By grilling the fruit, the skin and soft flesh caramelize to give it a sweeter flavor, and it releases its juices. Topped with the sharpness of the orange zest and the creamy Greek yogurt, it's a dreamy bit of heaven!

1 Arrange the nectarine segments on a hot BBQ grill or preheated ridged grill pan and cook until softened and slightly charred.

2 Serve on a plate with the yogurt, top with the orange zest and juice, and sprinkle with the chopped pistachios.

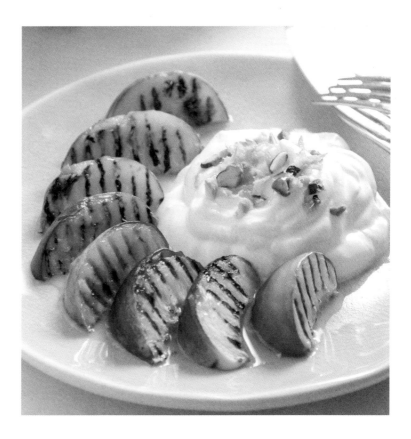

BANOFFEE ICE CREAM

SERVES ONE

1 banana, sliced and frozen

3 tbsp full-fat Greek OR Greek-style soy-based vegan yogurt

8 pecan halves, crushed

This is the easiest ice cream to make, and the healthiest! I'm a big fan of Greek yogurt, as it tends to have more protein and less sugar than regular yogurt. You do need to use frozen banana for this recipe, but it only takes a couple of hours at the most to freeze.

1 Place the frozen banana slices in a food processor with the Greek yogurt and blend until smooth, then fold three-quarters of the crushed pecans into the mixture.

2 You can serve this right away, but it will be quite soft. If you prefer a firmer texture, place it in the freezer for around 30 minutes, but keep checking and stirring so it freezes evenly and stays creamy.

3 Serve in your favorite glass or dish and sprinkle the remaining pecans over the top.

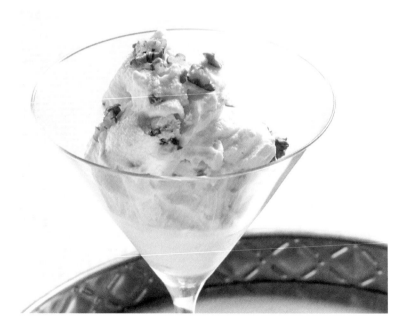

GOOD TO KNOW

This really is all about timing, so don't let your ice cream over-freeze, as it won't taste as good —keep checking!

KNICKERBOCKER GLORY

SERVES TWO

handful of raspberries

2 tsp chia seeds

handful of chopped pineapple

1 apple, diced

6 tbsp full-fat Greek OR Greek-style soy-based vegan yogurt

12 pecan halves, crushed

I used to love a knickerbocker glory when I was a child, and so I was determined to create a healthy version. For me, it's all about the contrasting textures of the fruit—it definitely makes the experience feel indulgent.

1 Blend the raspberries in a food processor or blender or mush them through a sieve until you have a really juicy pulp.

2 Place the raspberry pulp in a bowl and stir in the chia seeds, then set aside until they turn a little jellied. Place the pineapple in a blender and blend to a pulp.

3 In your favorite tall glass, create even layers with your ingredients, starting with the yogurt and finishing with fruit on top. Sprinkle with the crushed pecans and enjoy!

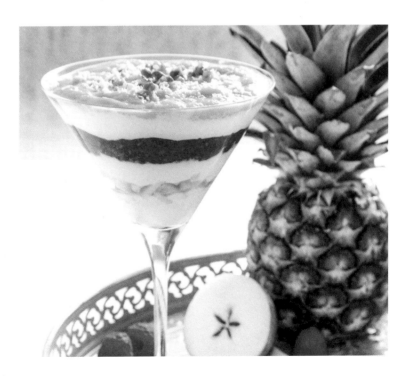

STRAWBERRY PARFAIT

SERVES ONE

handful of fresh strawberries, sliced

3 tbsp full-fat Greek OR Greek-style soy-based vegan yogurt

8 unsalted pistachios, chopped or crushed

Parfaits with yogurt and nuts are a tasty way to eat fresh strawberries without adding that unwanted topping of sugar! Pistachios are packed with antioxidants and nutrients and add a delicious crunch.

1 Place the strawberries in your favorite glass dish and mix in the yogurt. Top with those all-important pistachio nuts and enjoy!

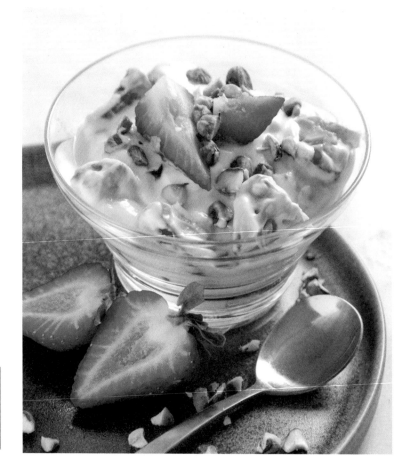

GOOD TO KNOW

Try to use ripe strawberries, as they are naturally sweeter and more flavorful.

STRAWBERRY ICE CREAM

SERVES TWO

handful of frozen strawberries

handful of frozen banana slices

½ serving (1 scoop; 40ml) of The Six Pack Revolution Strawberry Cream Sensation Post Workout Smoothie

2 tbsp full-fat Greek yogurt OR Greek-style soy-based vegan yogurt

12 cashew nuts

a generous ⅓ cup (100ml) unsweetened almond milk

2 fresh strawberries, sliced, to garnish

The Six Pack Revolution Strawberry Cream Sensation Post Workout Smoothie enhances both the flavor and creaminess of this delicious no-fuss ice cream. It's so easy to make and is perfect served with fresh strawberries on a summer's day.

1 Place the frozen fruit, smoothie powder, yogurt, cashews, and almond milk in a blender and blend to a smooth consistency.

2 Transfer the mixture to a freezer container and freeze for 3–4 hours, stirring every 45 minutes.

3 Serve with a scattering of fresh strawberries.

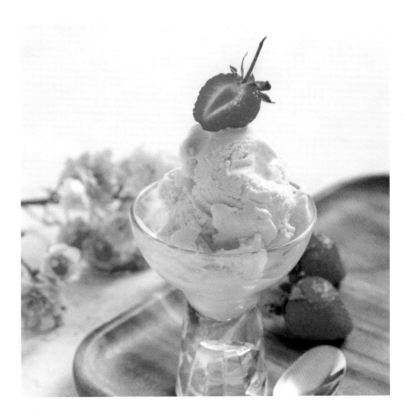

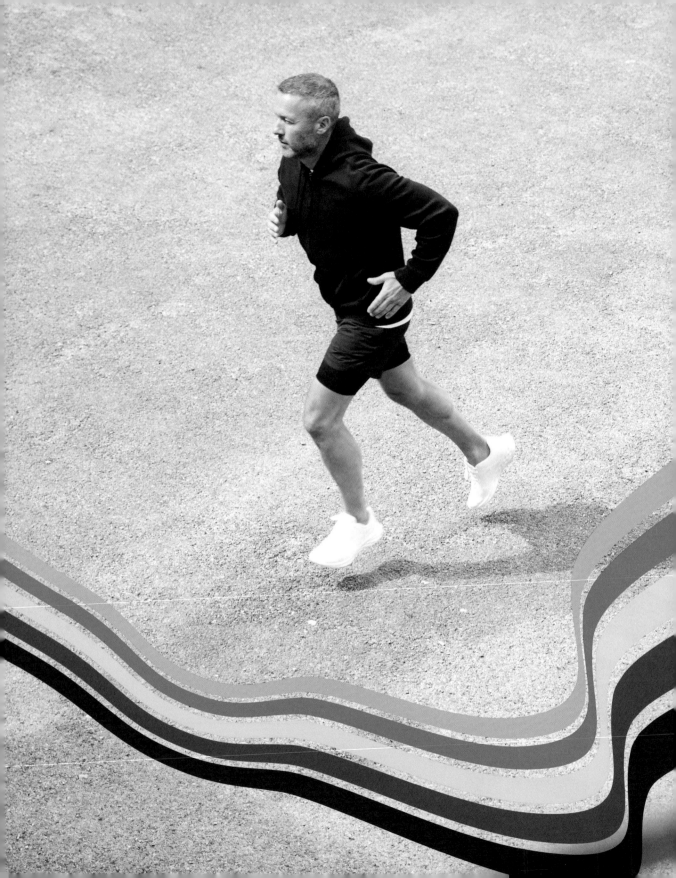

TRANSFORM BODY & MIND

Chapter Three

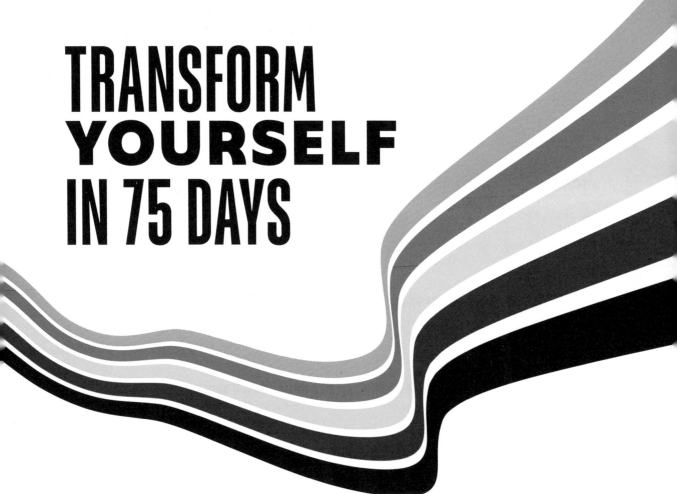

TRANSFORM YOURSELF IN 75 DAYS

The Ultimate 75 Day Transformation Plan is about combining nutrition and movement to create a positive balance in your life. On the following pages, I have designed 11 physical challenges for you to choose from. Perform at least two a week, starting with a warm up and ending with a cool down. Feel free to do more, if you like, but always include at least one rest day in every week, too. I promise you will notice transformative results.

A POSITIVE MINDSET

Creating positivity is the key to dealing with all the internal and external pressures of modern life, and not letting them overwhelm you. Then you can unlock your full potential.

HIGH FIVE TO ACCEPTANCE

Life is a roller-coaster ride, with ups and downs that are often beyond your control. Accepting that fact and dealing with issues head on will prevent you from giving up at the first hurdle.

FLEX YOUR GROWTH MUSCLES

Believe. Learn. Adapt. Setbacks are merely stepping-stones to your own success story.

PUMP UP THE POSITIVE TALK

That voice in your head—make it a friend and create a habit of positive self-talk, as this will build self-confidence and inner strength. Replace self-doubt with empowering affirmations.

EMBRACE CHANGE, UNLOCK RESILIENCE

When you step out of your comfort zone with arms wide open and welcome change with excitement, it's the path to personal growth and development. Resilience flourishes when you're adaptable and fearlessly embracing new experiences.

CHANGE YOUR MORNING ROUTINE

Wake up early, make your bed, stretch, exercise, and rehydrate. These small changes can positively affect the start of every day and, from here, watch your whole life transform.

FIND YOUR KIND

Surround yourself with like-minded individuals who can offer support, understanding, and motivation as you work on becoming a better you. In an environment of shared goals and aspirations, you'll find a sanctuary of collaborative coaching and inspiration.

SLEEP IS YOUR INVISIBLE ALLY

Quality sleep plays an integral role in mood regulation, stress reduction, and the ability to cope with life's challenges. In the quiet embrace of slumber, the mind calms, muscles recover, and the whole body grows stronger, ready to take on tomorrow's physical and mental challenges successfully.

THE PAST DOES NOT EXIST

It's only a memory. Don't look back, unless it's to reminisce about a happy time or to see how far you've come. Any regrets? Remember, you made the best choice at the time with the knowledge you had. Be at peace with it and move on.

THE FUTURE DOES NOT EXIST

It's only your imagination. Therefore, make sure you imagine the best future possible!

"THE BEST WAY TO INVEST IN YOUR FUTURE IS TO BELIEVE YOU ARE CAPABLE OF ANYTHING YOU PUT YOUR MIND TO"

SCOTT HARRISON

FIT FOR LIFE

The Six Pack Revolution provides a transformative journey that goes beyond appearances—it promises to make you fit for life. Embracing physical fitness will help you unlock a world of boundless energy and find a more positive perspective on so many things as you realize a stronger, more authentic self. As you shed excess pounds, your immune system thrives, mental clarity sharpens, and confidence soars with each fitness goal smashed. Eating healthily and exercising regularly can lead to clearer skin, better sleep, and improved hydration, which all contribute to a more vibrant and radiant life! Let's dive deeper into these amazing benefits:

LONG-TERM FAT LOSS

Fad diets and extreme exercise may offer temporary results, but for lasting changes, consistency and sustainability are key. What works is regular exercise, combined with a balanced diet, which is why this book gives you delicious recipes as well as a selection of eight proven challenges that you can easily do at home.

ARMOR UP

Regular exercise is your secret weapon to boost immunity. It sends those immune cells marching through your body, which are your first line of defense against infections and illnesses. It also reduces inflammation, which can lower the risk of developing chronic diseases.

BOOST YOUR MENTAL MOJO

Exercise is the ultimate mood-lifter, as it results in the release of endorphins, which help boost your self-esteem, crush those anxieties, and promote feelings of well-being.

SUPERCHARGE YOUR HEALTH

Regular exercise slashes the risk of heart disease, type 2 diabetes, and even certain cancers. Active individuals also score much better health outcomes for longevity.

UNLEASH MOBILITY MAGIC

Exercise is your fountain of youth, as it keeps joints flexible, muscles strong, and prevents age-related decline in functional abilities. Studies also prove that exercise can protect you from falls as you age. So, embrace the power of fitness and improve your mobility.

FORGE A MIGHTY MINDSET

This is about developing a lifelong romance with strength and vitality! Consistency is key. Dig deep and go for it! Remember, exercise is good for your bone density, muscle tone, joints, posture, and emotional state and is a huge investment in your future.

POWER UP

When you get your body moving, your blood flows and delivers an oxygen-packed punch to your muscles and tissues, leading to a surge in energy levels. This increased energy helps you feel more alert and focused throughout the day.

"YOU HAVE A CHOICE . . . LET THE HARD STUFF BEAT YOU OR LET IT TEACH YOU!"

SCOTT HARRISON

WARM UP

It really is important to warm up gently before you exercise, as this will slowly raise your heart rate and body temperature, increasing blood flow to the muscles and helping prevent soreness and injury. Your warm-up should consist of dynamic stretches and movements, as these put your joints and muscles through a full range of motion that will increase your flexibility and prepare you for your main challenge.

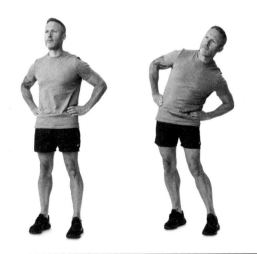

HIP CIRCLES
10 clockwise, 10 counter-clockwise

1 Stand tall, with your feet slightly wider than hip-width apart. Place your hands on your hips and engage your core.
2 Slowly and smoothly rotate your hips clockwise in a wide circle until you return to the starting position. Repeat counter-clockwise.

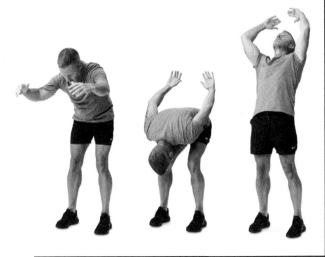

UP + OVERS
x 10

1 Stand tall, with your arms by your sides, core engaged, and knees slightly soft to avoid the legs locking.
2 Bend forward from the hips and allow the arms to hang heavy.
3 Slowly roll up to standing position and bring the arms up above the head.
4 Keeping the arms extended and pushing the pelvis forward, lean back to stretch even farther.
5 Swing back down and up again, repeating the full range of motion.

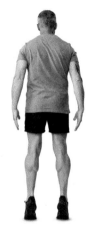

CALF RAISES
x 10

1 Stand tall, with your feet shoulder-width apart, toes pointing forward, and arms by your side. Engage your core.
2 Raise your heels slowly so that you come up onto your tiptoes. Keep your legs straight and ensure the knees don't lock. Feel the stretch in your calf muscles and hold for 2 seconds.
3 Slowly lower your heels back to the floor, returning to the starting position.

DEEP SQUAT STRETCH

Hold for 20 seconds

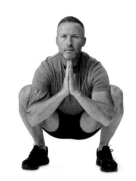

1 Stand tall, with your feet very slightly turned out and placed a little wider than hip-width apart, and come into a low squat position.
2 Place your palms together and, trying to keep your feet flat on the floor, press your elbows into the inside of your knees and gently push out.

ARM CIRCLES

10 forward, 10 backward

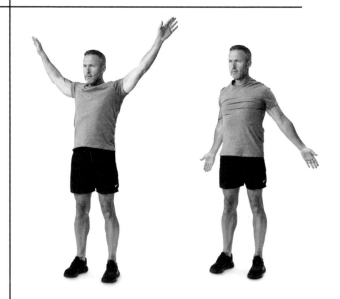

1 Stand tall, with your feet shoulder-width apart, shoulders relaxed, and core engaged. Raise and extend your arms out to the side.
2 Slowly rotate your arms forward in big circles.
3 Complete a set of 10 forward circles, then repeat the same movements in a backward direction.

KNEE RAISES

Hold for 10 seconds

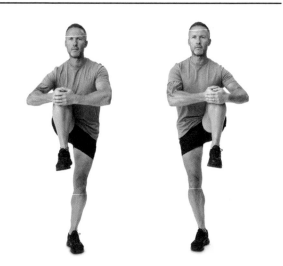

1 Stand tall, with your feet hip-width apart. Pick a point directly in front of you to focus your gaze on and find your balance.
2 With your left foot firmly planted on the ground, raise your right knee and use your hands to hug it to the chest and hold, then lower and repeat on the opposite side.

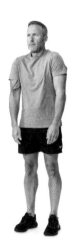
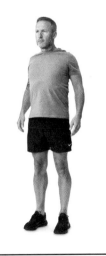

ROLLING SHOULDERS
10 forward, 10 backward

1 Stand tall, with your feet shoulder-width apart, arms by your side, and shoulders relaxed.
2 Lift your shoulders up to your ears, keeping the neck and head relaxed, and roll the shoulders forward and down.
3 Repeat the same movement in a backward direction.

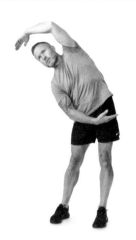
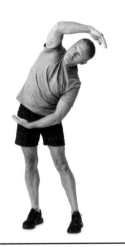

SIDE STRETCH
x 10 on each side

1 Stand tall, with your feet shoulder-width apart and arms by your side.
2 Raise your left arm so that the elbow is in line with your ear and bend the arm over your head.
3 Gently lean to the right so that your left arm extends over and increases the stretch.
4 Keeping the left elbow in line with your left ear, reach the opposite arm across the abdomen.
5 Repeat on the opposite side.

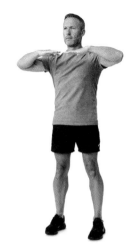
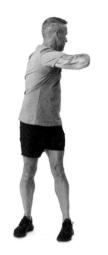

TORSO TWISTS
x 10 on each side

1 Stand tall, with your feet shoulder-width apart, and raise your elbows to shoulder height, with your hands in front of your chest. Keep the shoulders relaxed and core engaged.
2 Gently twist your torso to the left until you feel the stretch and then gently rotate back through the center and twist to the right.

COOL
DOWN

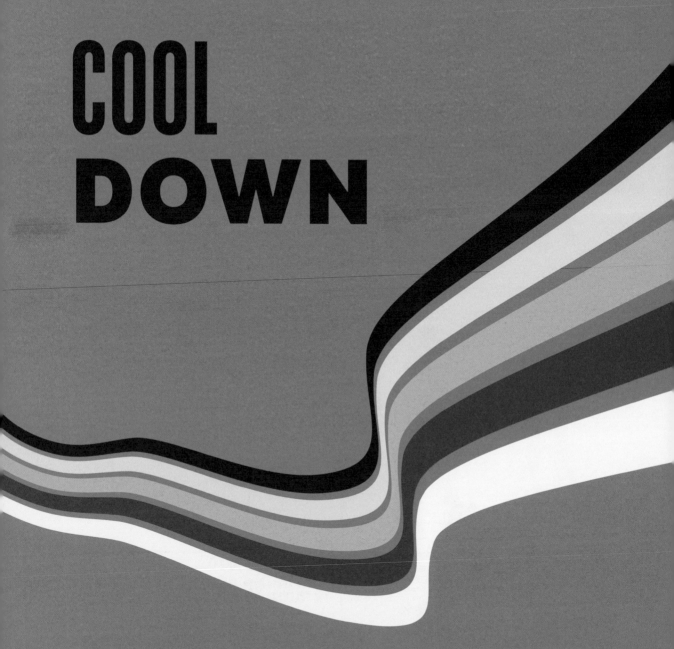

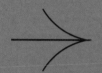

It is just as important to stretch AFTER every challenge, as this will slowly lower your heart rate and return your muscles to a resting state. This also helps avoid soreness and injuries after exercising.

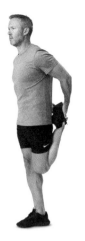

QUAD STRETCH
Hold for 10 seconds

1   Stand tall with your feet hip-width apart and pick a point directly in front of you to focus your gaze on —this will help you find your balance. You can also use a chair or wall for support, if you need to.
2   Raise your left foot toward your left buttock and grasp your ankle with your left hand.
3   Keep your knees together and push your hips forward slightly to find the stretch. Hold for 10 seconds, then lower the foot to the ground and return to the starting position. Repeat on the opposite side.

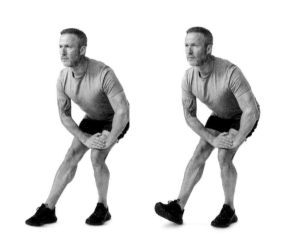

HAMSTRING TO CALF STRETCH
Hold for 10 seconds

1   Stand tall, with your feet shoulder-width apart.
2   Step your right leg forward and, keeping the left foot planted flat on the floor, extend your right leg in front of you, heel to the ground. Push your bottom back and bend the left leg to support you; feel the stretch in the hamstring. Rest your hands just above your bent knee to help you balance and hold for 10 seconds.
3   Lift the toes to stretch into the calf and hold again, then return to the starting position. Repeat with the opposite leg.

This exercise should be avoided if you have any ankle, knee, or hip injuries, where external rotation is restricted or painful.

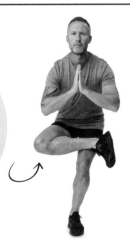

STANDING PIGEON
Hold for 10 seconds

1   Stand tall, with your feet shoulder-width apart, toes pointing forward, and find your balance. You can also use a chair or wall, if you need to.
2   Planting your left foot firmly into the ground, lift the right foot and place it just above the knee of the supporting leg. Lower your hips back and down into a gentle squat and bring your hands together in a prayer position (they will help you balance).
3   Hold for 10 seconds and then return to the starting position and repeat on the opposite side.

WRIST STRETCH
Hold for 10 seconds

1 Stand tall, with your feet shoulder-width apart, and lift both arms straight out in front of you at shoulder height.
2 Point the fingers down toward the floor and hold, feeling the stretch in the top of the wrist and forearms. Hold for 10 seconds.
3 Point the fingers up toward the sky, slightly lowering the arms and feeling the stretch in your lower wrist and forearms. Hold for 10 seconds.

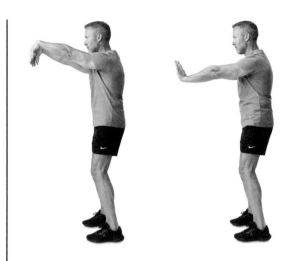

CHEST STRETCH
Hold for 10 seconds

1 Stand tall, with your feet shoulder-width apart, shoulders relaxed, and place the palms of your hands on the small of your back, with fingertips pointing down so they meet in the center of your spine, the elbows pointing behind you.
2 Squeeze the shoulder blades together to feel the stretch across your chest. Hold for 10 seconds.

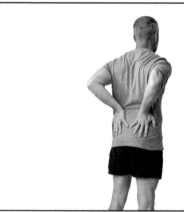

BICEP STRETCH
Hold for 10 seconds

1 Stand tall, with your feet shoulder-width apart. Extend your arms down in front of you and clench your fists.
2 Keeping the arms straight, take them back directly behind you, keeping the fists clenched and pushing the fists up and away. Bend slightly at the hips as the arms reach behind. Hold for 10 seconds.

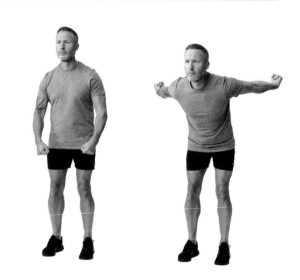

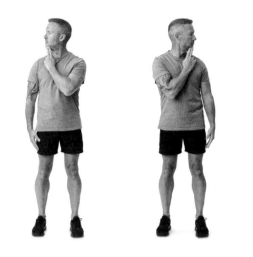

NECK STRETCH
Hold for 10 seconds

1 Stand tall, shoulders relaxed and feet shoulder-width apart.
2 Keep your chin parallel to the floor and slowly turn your head to the right. Gently apply a little pressure to the chin to extend the stretch but be careful not to strain the neck. Hold for 10 seconds.
3 Repeat on the opposite side.

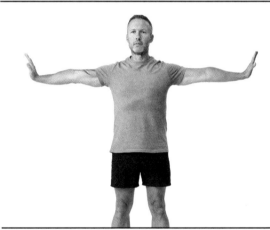

PUSH THE WALLS
Hold for 10 seconds

1 Stand tall, with your feet shoulder-width apart, engage your core, and extend your arms out at shoulder height so that your fingers point up toward the sky.
2 Push out, as if against a wall, until you feel the stretch through your arms and across your back.

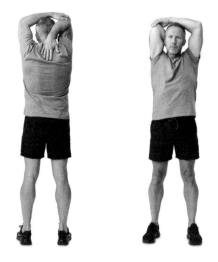

TRICEP STRETCH
Hold for 10 seconds

1 Stand tall, with your feet shoulder-width apart and shoulders relaxed.
2 Take one arm straight up and bend at the elbow so that the palm of the hand reaches between your shoulder blades, toward the centre of your back, and the elbow points toward the sky.
3 Raise your other hand and, holding the elbow, apply gentle pressure to extend the stretch. Hold for 10 seconds, then return to the starting position and repeat on the opposite side.

CROSS-ARM STRETCH
Hold for 10 seconds

1 Stand tall, with your feet shoulder-width apart. Lift one arm and extend it across the body, keeping the elbow raised.
2 Use your other hand or arm to hold the extended arm at the elbow and apply gentle pressure to feel the stretch. Hold for 10 seconds, then return to the starting position.
3 Repeat on the opposite side.

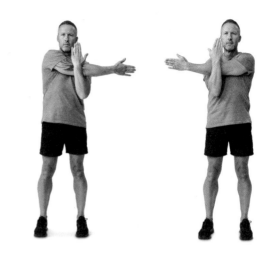

CHILD POSE
Hold for 60 seconds

1 Come down onto the floor on all fours. Sit back onto your heels and spread your knees wide.
2 Pressing your hips down and back, lower your body so that your tummy rests between your thighs and place your forehead on the floor.
3 Extend both arms out in front of you, palms down and fingers splayed, and feel the stretch and a feeling of calm. Hold for 60 seconds, breathing deeply in through the nose and out through the mouth.

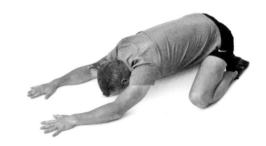

So, now that you know how to warm up and cool down, let's move on to the challenges. How many breaks you take is up to you, but I encourage you to push yourself. You will be surprised at how quickly your fitness improves when combining these challenges with the nutrition of The Six Pack Revolution—enjoy!

EXERCISE CHALLENGES

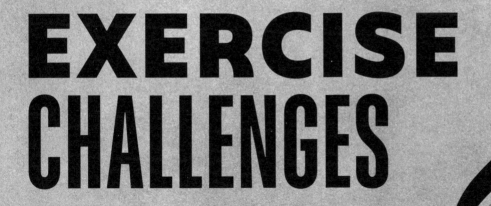

CHALLENGE 1

PRESSED FOR TIME

- This is all about short bursts of exercise and is a super-speedy and efficient way to get your challenge in—if you're "pressed for time," you'll be done in 20 minutes and feeling the fat-burning benefits for the next 24 hours!

- Perform each exercise in the sequence for 40 seconds, then rest for 20 seconds before moving on to the next.

- Perform the entire sequence for 3 rounds, resting for 1 minute between each round.

FAST FEET

1 **START POSITION:** Stand tall, with your feet hip-width apart.
2 Run in place—try to land lightly on the balls of your feet and keep your knees low while pumping your arms.
3 Keep your core engaged and legs moving fast.

SQUATS

1 **START POSITION:** Stand tall, with your feet shoulder-width apart and your weight in your heels.
2 Push your bottom back and bend your knees until your thighs are parallel to the ground. Keep your back straight and chest up.
3 Drive through your heels to stand up straight. Squeeze your glutes and keep your core tight as you perform the movement.

SKATER HOPS

1 **START POSITION:** Move to the left of your space and squat slightly.
2 Jump to the right, landing on your right foot, and take your left foot across and behind.
3 Jump back across to the left—this time, the right foot crosses behind the left as we repeat the move on the opposite side.

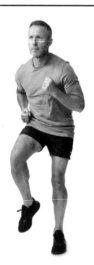

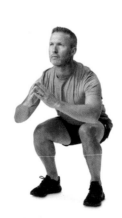

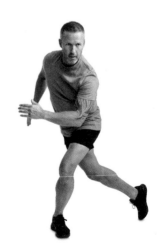

HIGH KNEES

1 **START POSITION:** Stand tall, with your feet hip-width apart and hands at waist height, palms facing down.
2 Run on the spot, bringing your knees up toward your hands, as high as possible.

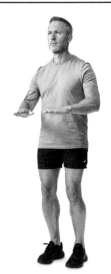

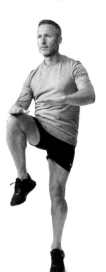

PUSH-UPS

Push-ups can be challenging, especially for anyone with wrist, elbow, or lower back pain. However, you can also perform them with your knees on the floor and body at a 45-degree angle, as this places less pressure on these areas. Alternatively, push against a wall.

1 **START POSITION:** High plank—hands flat on the floor about shoulder-width apart, wrists under shoulders, body in one long, straight line, and toes curled.
2 Keeping your core engaged and body in one long line, bend your arms and lower yourself as close to the floor as you can. Your elbows should be behind your shoulders at about a 45-degree angle.
3 Push back up to the start position and repeat.

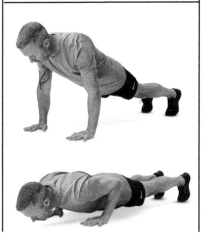

SQUAT KICKS

1 **START POSITION:** Stand with your feet shoulder-width apart and your weight in your heels.
2 Push the bottom back and bend your knees until your thighs are parallel to the ground, keeping the back straight and chest up.
3 Drive through your heels to stand back up, lift the knee, and kick one leg straight out in front of you. Squeeze your glutes and keep your core tight as you return the leg to the ground and move into the next squat, kicking with the opposite leg, and then repeat.

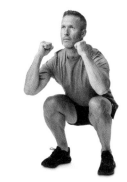

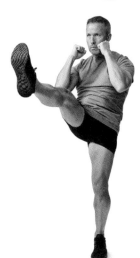

CHALLENGE 2

BUILD WITH BODYWEIGHT

- When you don't have access to weights or don't have time to get to the gym, your own bodyweight provides a great alternative and is all you need to really work those muscles. No equipment is required, and you can simply adjust the tempo of your challenge to suit your ability and preferences for the day.

- Perform each exercise in sequence, resting between sets as needed (15–20 seconds).

PUSH-UPS

3 x 20 Sets

1 **START POSITION:** High plank —hands flat on the floor about shoulder-width apart, wrists under shoulders, body in one long, straight line, and toes curled.
2 Keeping your core engaged and body in one long line, bend your arms and lower yourself as close to the floor as you can. Your elbows should be behind your shoulders at about a 45-degree angle.
3 Push back up to the start position and repeat.

PLANK ROTATION KICK RIGHT AND LEFT

4 x 10 Sets

1 **START POSITION:** High plank—hands flat on the floor about shoulder-width apart, wrists under shoulders, body in one long, straight line, and toes curled. Ensure your abs are engaged and your glutes are tight.
2 Bring your right foot under your body, toward the left. At the same time, reach your left hand to touch your right foot, balancing on your right arm and left leg. Repeat 10 times.
3 Perform steps 1 and 2 on the other side.

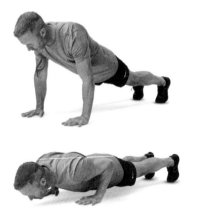

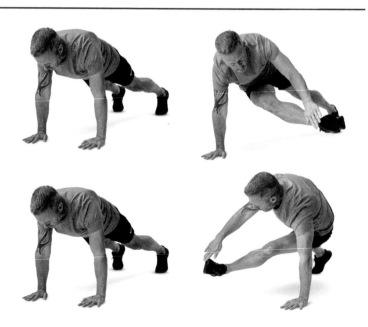

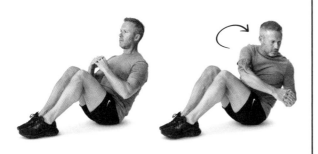

RUSSIAN TWISTS
4 x 20 Sets

1 **START POSITION:** Sit on the floor with your legs out in front of you, knees bent and heels flat.
2 Keeping your core engaged, lean back slightly so that your body and legs form a V-shape.
3 Keeping the core strong and knees straight, twist your torso from side to side. The movement is all focused in the abdomen—try not to let the knees move too much.

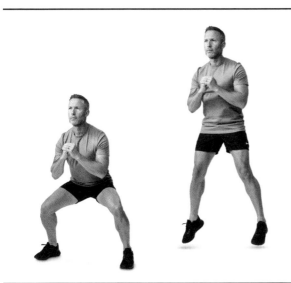

SQUAT JUMPS
4 x 20 Sets

1 **START POSITION:** Stand with your feet slightly wider than hip-width apart.
2 Push your bottom back and bend your knees until your thighs are parallel to the ground, keeping your back straight and chest up.
3 Drive through your heels and jump up into the air as high as you can, straightening out your legs. Ensure the knees are soft as you land and repeat.

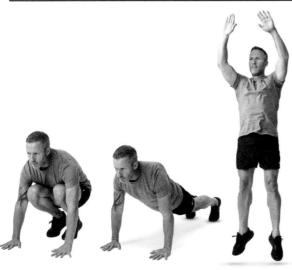

BURPEES
3 x 10 Sets

1 **START POSITION:** Stand with your feet shoulder-width apart.
2 Bend your knees and reach forward to place your hands on the floor.
3 Kick both legs straight out behind you into a high plank position.
4 Hop your legs back under your body and jump straight up into the air, reaching your arms overhead.
5 Land with your knees slightly bent, then return to the start position and repeat.

CHALLENGE 3

HIGH-ENERGY HIIT

- High-Energy HIIT will fire up those endorphins, boost your metabolism, and build strength—giving you a complete full-body challenge.

- Perform each exercise for 45 seconds, then rest for 15–20 seconds. Work in sequence and complete the whole challenge 3 times, resting for 1 minute between each round.

- **EXTRA CHALLENGE:** Perform the whole challenge for 4 rounds.

HIGH KNEES

1 **START POSITION:** Stand tall, with your feet hip-width apart and hands at waist height, palms facing down.
2 Run on the spot, bringing your knees up toward your hands, as high as possible.
3 Keep your chest lifted and drive off the balls of your feet as you launch into the next step.

STANDING OBLIQUE CRUNCHES LEFT AND RIGHT

1 **START POSITION:** Stand tall, with your feet hip-width apart, hands placed at your temples, and elbows wide.
2 Lift your left knee up while lowering the right elbow down to meet it.
3 Repeat on the other side.

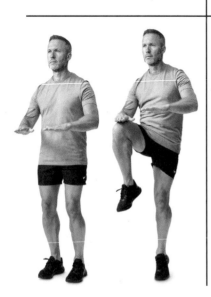 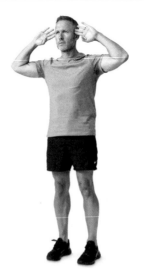 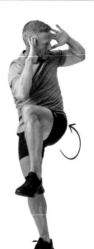 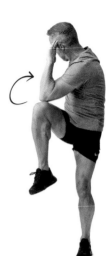

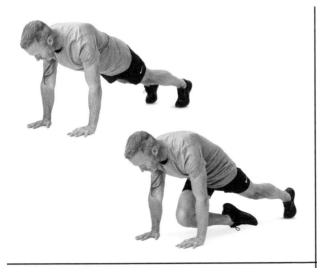

MOUNTAIN CLIMBERS

1 **START POSITION:** High plank—hands flat on the floor about shoulder-width apart, wrists under shoulders, body in one long, straight line, and toes curled. Ensure your abs are engaged and your glutes are tight.
2 Lift your right foot, bringing your knee in toward your chest as far as you can.
3 Replace your right foot on the ground and immediately lift your left foot, bringing your knee in toward the chest as far as you can.
4 Keep your hips down and continue switching legs, as if you're running in place.

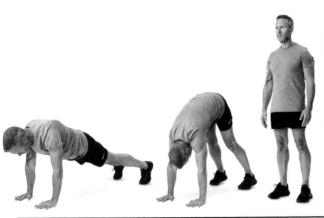

INCH WORMS

1 **START POSITION:** Stand tall, with your feet hip-width apart.
2 Bend forward from the hip and reach your hands toward the floor in front of you. Walk the hands out into a high plank position.
3 Walk your hands back toward your feet and return to standing, slowly straightening your back, one vertebra at a time.

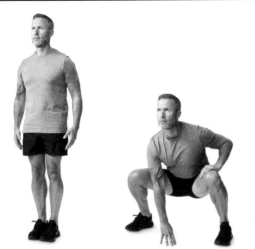

PLYOMETRIC SIDE SQUATS

1 **START POSITION:** Stand with your feet together.
2 Step to the right, push your bottom back, and bend your knees until your thighs are parallel to the ground. Keeping the back straight and chest up, tap the floor with your left fingertips.
3 Drive through the heels to return to an upright position, and step to the opposite side as you go into another squat. This time, tap the floor with your right fingertips.
4 Keep moving at a comfortable pace.

CHALLENGE 4

HIT THE FLOOR FOR THE CORE

- We all love to work those abs, and this floor challenge will give your core an all-around blitz. Add this one to another challenge when you're in the mood to give yourself an extra push.

- Perform 20 reps of each exercise in sequence, resting as needed in between, then repeat the whole sequence for 3 rounds.

MARCHING GLUTE BRIDGE

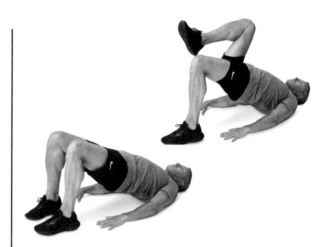

1 **START POSITION:** Lie on your back, with your knees bent, feet flat on the floor. Lift your hips and engage your glutes at the top.
2 Keeping your left knee bent and your hips still, lift your right foot off the floor.
3 Pause at the top, then slowly lower your right foot to the ground, but keep your hips lifted.
4 Repeat on alternating sides, keeping the hips lifted throughout.

SIDE PLANK DIPS

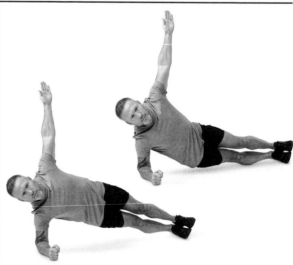

1 **START POSITION:** Start in a side plank position, resting on your right forearm. Stack your left foot on top of your right, keep your body in a straight line, and raise your left arm straight up.
2 Drop your hips toward the floor, then raise back higher than the starting position.
3 Repeat on the other side.

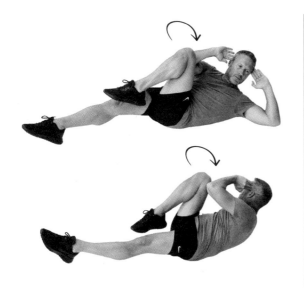

BICYCLE CRUNCHES

1 **START POSITION:** Lie on your back with your knees bent, feet lifted, and your hands lightly touching your temples.
2 Lift your shoulders to engage the core and keep your back flat against the floor—not arched.
3 Twist to bring your right elbow to your left knee as you straighten your right leg.
4 Alternate sides with control.

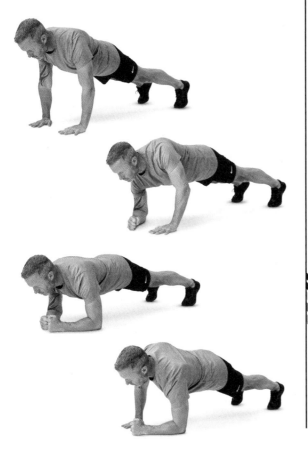

PLANK UP AND DOWN

1 **START POSITION:** High plank—hands flat on the floor about shoulder-width apart, wrists under shoulders, body in one long, straight line, and toes curled. Ensure your abs are engaged and your glutes are tight.
2 Bend your right arm to bring the elbow and forearm to the floor and clench your fists as you bring your left arm down to a forearm plank, hands meeting in the middle.
3 Push back up, first with your right arm, then with your left arm to the start position, replacing the hands where the elbows were on the floor.
4 Repeat, leading with alternating arms.

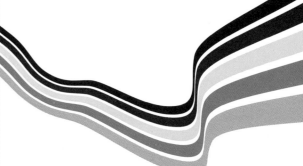

BEAR PLANKS

1 **START POSITION:** Start on your hands and knees in tabletop position, wrists in line with your shoulders and knees in line with your hips.
2 Curl your toes and lift your knees off the ground so you are hovering on your hands and toes. Keep your back flat and use your core to balance.
3 Slowly tap a hand on its opposite knee and repeat, alternating sides.
4 Keep your hips steady and core strong and try not to twist your body.

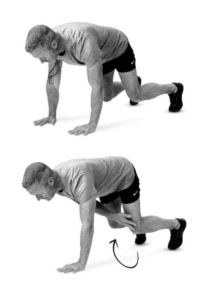

DEAD BUGS

1 **START POSITION:** Lie on your back, with your arms raised toward the ceiling. Bring your legs up into tabletop position, knees bent at a 90-degree angle and in line with your hips.
2 Slowly extend your left leg out straight while simultaneously dropping your right arm overhead. Keep both raised a few inches from the ground.
3 Bring your arm and leg back to the starting position and repeat, alternating the opposite arm and leg each time.

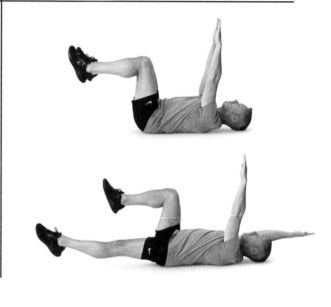

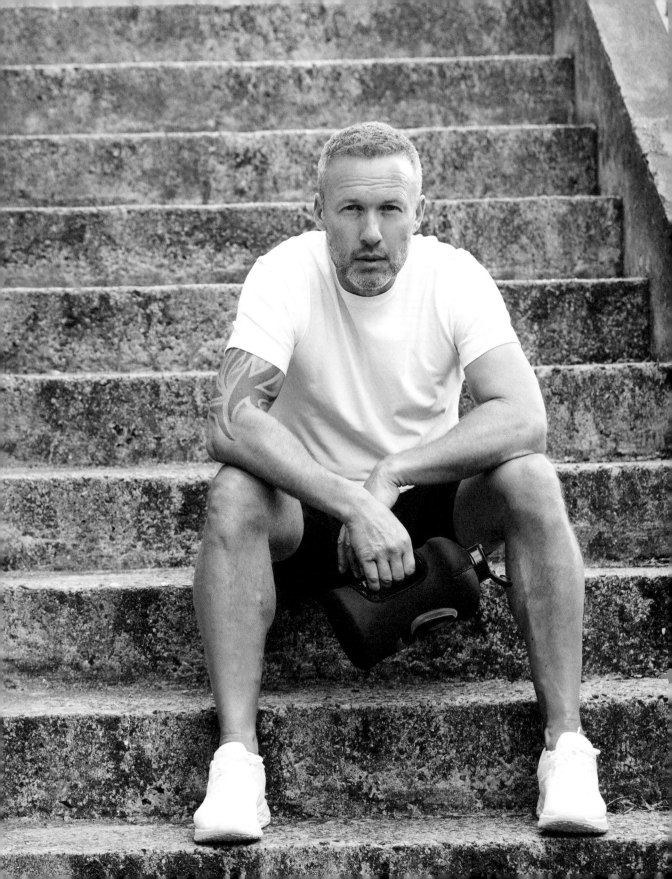

CHALLENGE 5

FULL BODY FOCUS

- This challenge will work all of your major muscle groups, hitting the arms, legs, and core—testing your balance, stability, and coordination.

- Perform each exercise in sequence for 1 minute, with short rests in between. Complete as many rounds as you can in the time you have available.

PRESS UPS

1. **START POSITION:** High plank —hands flat on the floor about shoulder-width apart, wrists under shoulders, body in one long, straight line, and toes curled.
2. Keeping your core engaged, bend your arms and lower yourself as close to the floor as you can. Ensure the elbows, behind your shoulders, are at about a 45-degree angle.
3. Push back up to the start position and repeat.

PLANK JACKS

1. **START POSITION:** High plank with your feet together—hands flat on the floor about shoulder-width apart, wrists under shoulders, body in one long, straight line, and toes curled.
2. Engage your core and jump both feet straight out in opposite directions.
3. Jump the legs back in and repeat.

SQUAT THRUSTS

1. **START POSITION:** High plank with your feet together—hands flat on the floor about shoulder-width apart, wrists under shoulders, body in one long, straight line, and toes curled.
2. Jump your feet to bring your knees in to your chest, then jump your feet back to a high plank position, and repeat.

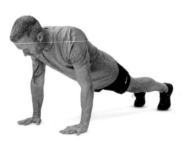
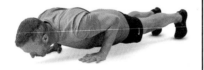
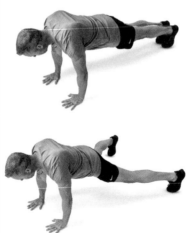
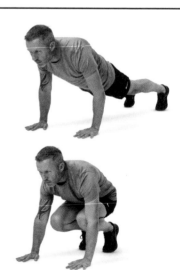

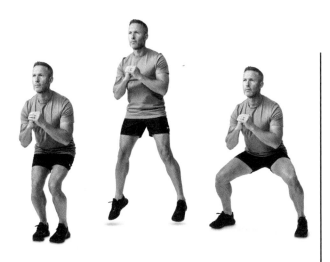

SQUAT JACKS

1 **START POSITION:** Stand tall with feet together, core engaged, and hands clasped at your chest.
2 Jump both feet out and sit back into a small squat, keeping the chest high and shoulders relaxed.
3 Jump your feet back together to return to standing and repeat.

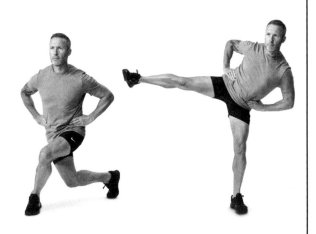

CURTSY LUNGE WITH SIDE KICK

1 **START POSITION:** Stand tall, feet hip-width apart, with hands on hips.
2 Step your right leg diagonally behind your left leg and bend your knees to lower into a lunge.
3 Push through your left heel to stand and kick your right leg out to the opposite side.
4 Bring your right leg down and back to the start position, then repeat on the opposite side.

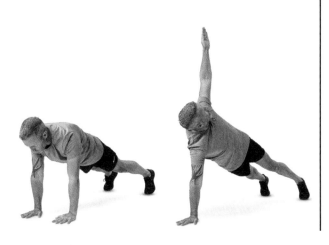

PLANK WITH T ROTATION

1 **START POSITION:** High plank—hands flat on the floor about shoulder-width apart, wrists under shoulders, body in one long, straight line, and toes curled.
2 Rotate your entire body to the right into a side plank so that your shoulders are in line with your right wrist.
3 Extend your left arm to the ceiling, looking up at your pointed fingertips and keeping your hips lifted.
4 Return to the center position, then repeat on the opposite side.

CHALLENGE 6

LET'S TALK ABOUT LEGS

- Yes, we have to, because our legs contain the largest muscles in the body and we use them every day, so they need to be strong. However, as we focus on the lower body here, you'll also be working the core for stability and balance.

- Perform each exercise in sequence for 40 seconds, then rest for 20 seconds. At the end of each round, rest back into child pose for 1 minute. Repeat for a total of 3 rounds.

SQUAT JACKS

1 **START POSITION:** Stand tall, with your feet together and hands clasped at the chest.
2 Jump your feet out and sit back into a small squat, keeping the chest high.
3 Jump your feet back together to return to standing and repeat.

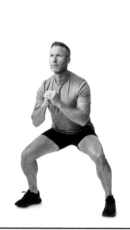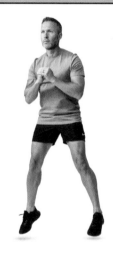

SIDE-STEP SQUATS

1 **START POSITION:** Start in a standing position, with feet together and hands by your side.
2 Take a wide step with your right foot, so your feet are just wider than shoulder-width apart.
3 Push your weight through the heels and bend your knees to lower into a squat, keeping your chest up and back straight.
4 Straighten your knees and bring your foot back to the starting position.
5 Repeat on the left side and then keep alternating.

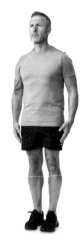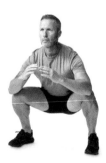

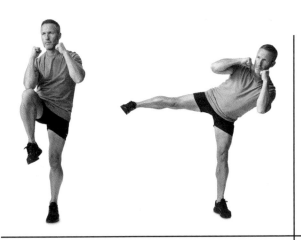

HIGH KNEE TO SIDE KICK

1 START POSITION: Stand tall with your feet together, hands raised, and fists clenched.
2 Bring your right knee up toward your chest. Then, with the same leg, kick out to the side.
3 Repeat on the left side and then keep alternating sides.

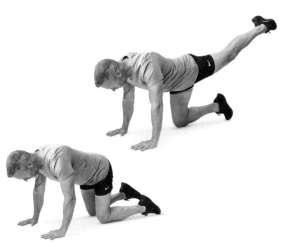

SINGLE LEG KICKBACKS

1 START POSITION: Start on all fours with your knees under your hips and hands under your shoulders.
2 Lift your right leg and flex your foot as you kick it back behind you, straightening your leg and squeezing your glutes.
3 Return to the start position and repeat on the left side and then keep alternating sides.

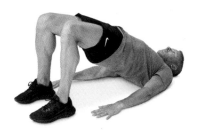
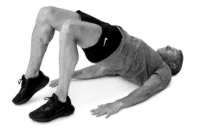

GLUTE BRIDGE WITH ALTERNATING CALF RAISE

1 START POSITION: Lie on your back, with your knees bent and feet flat on the floor. Lift your hips, engaging your glutes at the top.
2 While the hips are raised, come onto tiptoes on your right foot and hold for one second, then lower and come onto tiptoes on your left foot.
3 Keep alternating sides like you are walking.

CHALLENGE 7

GET TO THE CORE

- A strong core isn't just about the crunches, as the central part of your body needs to work in harmony, whether you're on a sport's field or carrying the groceries. Perform 2 rounds and your core will humming, 3 and it will be singing.

- Work for 45 seconds, then rest for 15 seconds.

- Repeat for a total of 2 rounds, resting for 1 minute between rounds for a great time-saving challenge.

- Repeat for a total of 3 rounds, if you'd like an extra challenge.

ALTERNATING SINGLE LEG RAISES

1 **START POSITION:** Lie on your back, with your knees either bent or straight out in front of you. Inhale.
2 As you exhale, keeping your back pushed into the floor, raise one leg straight up and flex the foot. Hold for a second, then lower.
3 Repeat with the other leg and then keep alternating sides.

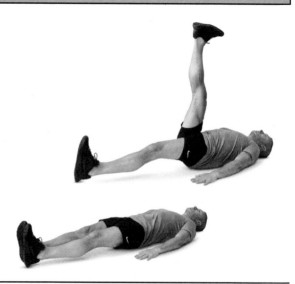

BUTTERFLY GLUTE BRIDGES

1 **START POSITION:** Lie on your back, with your knees bent. Bring your feet together and let your knees fall out to the side.
2 Squeeze your glutes and push your hips up toward the sky, then lower with control and repeat.

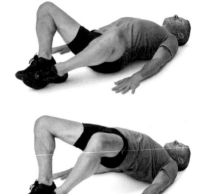

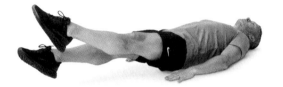

FLUTTERKICKS

1 **START POSITION:** Lie on your back, with your legs straight out in front, hands on the floor by y our side.
2 Engaging the core and keeping your back pushed into the floor, raise your feet off the floor and "flutter" your legs up and down, as if swimming through water.

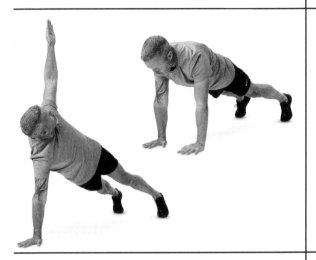

PLANK WITH T ROTATION

1 **START POSITION:** High plank—hands flat on the floor about shoulder-width apart, wrists under shoulders, body in one long, straight line, and toes curled.
2 Rotate your entire body to the right into a side plank so that your shoulders are in line with your right wrist.
3 Extend your left arm to the ceiling, looking up at your pointed fingertips and keeping your hips lifted.
4 Return to the center position, then repeat on the opposite side.

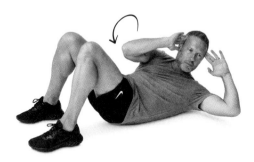

OBLIQUE CRUNCHES

1 **START POSITION:** Lie on your back, with your knees bent, hands lightly touching your temples, with elbows wide.
2 Engaging the core and keeping the lower back pushed into the floor, lift the upper body as you reach the right elbow to the left knee.
3 Keeping the arms wide, alternate sides as you repeat.

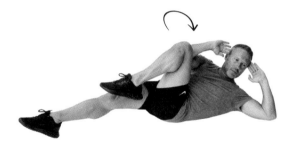

BICYCLE CRUNCHES

1 **START POSITION:** Lie on your back, with knees bent, hands lightly touching your temples.
2 Lift the shoulders and twist to bring your right elbow to your left knee as you straighten your right leg.
3 Alternate each side with control.

CHALLENGE 8

TIME FOR TABATA

- Tabata is another style of High-Intensity Interval Training—20 seconds of maximum effort, followed by 10 seconds of rest. Give it all you've got for 20 seconds, and you know you've got a brief rest before you go again.

- Perform each exercise for 20 seconds, then rest for 10 seconds. Repeat each pair for a total of 4 minutes before moving on to the next pair. Complete as many rounds as you dare!

JUMPING JACKS

1. **START POSITION:** Stand tall, with your feet together and hands by your sides.
2. Jump up, spread your feet, and bring both hands together above your head.
3. Jump again and return to the starting position.
4. Repeat until the time is complete.

JUMP SQUATS

1. **START POSITION:** Stand with your feet slightly wider than hip-width apart.
2. Push your bottom back and bend your knees until your thighs are parallel to the ground, keeping your back straight and chest up.
3. Drive through your heels and jump up into the air as high as you can, straightening out your legs. Ensure the knees are soft as you land and keep repeating.

EXERCISE PAIR 1

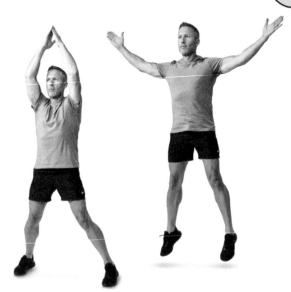
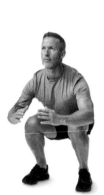
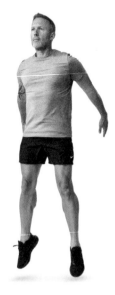

MOUNTAIN CLIMBERS

1 **START POSITION:** High plank—hands flat on the floor about shoulder-width apart, wrists under shoulders, body in one long, straight line, and toes curled. Ensure your abs are engaged and your glutes are tight.
2 Lift your right foot, bringing your knee in toward your chest as far as you can.
3 Replace the right foot on the ground and immediately lift the left foot, bringing your knee in toward the chest as far as you can.
4 Keep your hips down and continue switching legs, as if you're running in place.

SIDE-STEP SQUATS

1 **START POSITION:** Stand tall, with feet together and hands on your hips.
2 Step your right foot out, so your feet are just wider than shoulder-width apart.
3 Push your weight through the heels and bend your knees to lower into a squat, keeping your chest up and back straight.
4 Straighten your knees and bring your foot back to the starting position.
5 Repeat on the left and then keep alternating sides.

EXERCISE PAIR 2

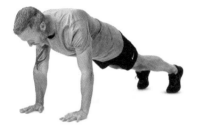
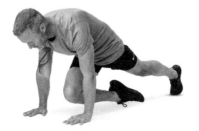
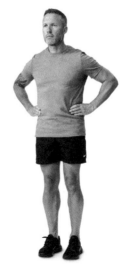
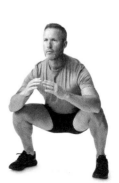

Make sure you view each challenge just like an obstacle course. Your job is simply to get from the beginning to the end. How many breaks you take is up to you, but push yourself.

SKATER HOPS

1 **START POSITION:** Move to the left of your space and squat slightly.
2 Jump to the right, landing on your right foot, and take your left foot across and behind.
3 Jump back across to the left, but this time the right foot crosses behind the left as we repeat the move on the opposite side.

MOUNTAIN CLIMBERS

1 **START POSITION:** High plank—hands flat on the floor about shoulder-width apart, wrists under shoulders, body in one long, straight line, and toes curled. Ensure your abs are engaged and your glutes are tight.
2 Lift your right foot, bringing your knee in toward your chest as far as you can.
3 Replace your right foot on the ground and immediately lift your left foot, bringing your knee in toward the chest.
4 Keeping the hips down, continue switching legs, as if you're running in place.

EXERCISE PAIR 3

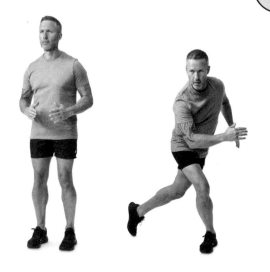

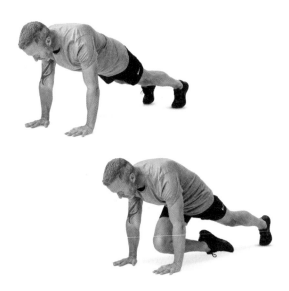

CHALLENGE 9

PYRAMIDS

- This challenge harnesses the power of a pyramid with 3 simple exercises that have maximum impact! It's quick and simple, can be done anywhere, and will stimulate your muscles to grow. I recommend you do it once a week.

- This is all about gradually increasing the reps at first and then reducing them:

- Perform 1 rep of each exercise, then 2, 3, 4, 5, 6, 7, 8, 9, 10

- Perform 10 reps of each exercise, then 9, 8, 7, 6, 5, 4, 3, 2, 1

CRUNCHES

1 **START POSITION:** Lie on your back, feet flat on the floor and hip-width apart, and knees bent. Place your arms across your chest or lightly touch your temples with your fingertips.
2 Inhale, then on the exhale, lift the upper body, keeping the head and neck relaxed.
3 Inhale as you return to the starting position.

PUSH-UPS

1 **START POSITION:** High plank —hands flat on the floor about shoulder-width apart, wrists under shoulders, body in one long, straight line, and toes curled.
2 Keeping your core engaged and body in one long line, bend your arms and lower yourself as close to the floor as you can. Your elbows should be behind your shoulders at about a 45-degree angle.
3 Push back up to the start position and repeat.

SQUATS

1 **START POSITION:** Stand tall, with your feet about shoulder-width apart and your weight in your heels.
2 Push your bottom back and bend your knees until your thighs are parallel to the ground. Keep your back straight and chest up.
3 Drive through your heels to stand up straight. Squeeze your glutes and keep your core tight as you perform the movement. Repeat.

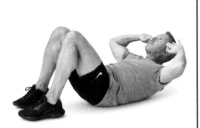

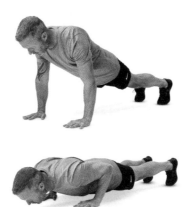

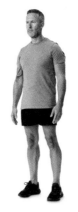

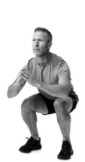

CHALLENGE 10

10 FOR 10

- Not one for the faint-hearted—this challenge will test the mind as well as the muscles. Try to keep going for the whole 10 rounds.

- Complete 10 reps of each exercise in sequence.

- Repeat for a total of 10 rounds—you can do it!

LUNGE WITH TOE TAP

1 **START POSITION:** Stand tall, feet hip-width apart and hands on hips.
2 Step your right leg diagonally behind your left leg and bend your knees to lower into a lunge. Tap the toe of the supporting leg with your right hand.
3 Push through your right heel to stand, then repeat on the opposite side and keep alternating.

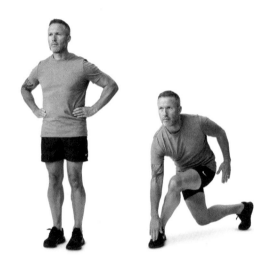

PLANK SHOULDER TAPS

1 **START POSITION:** High plank position, with your feet slightly wider than hip-width apart.
2 Keeping your core engaged and your hips as still as possible, tap each hand on the opposite shoulder and repeat.

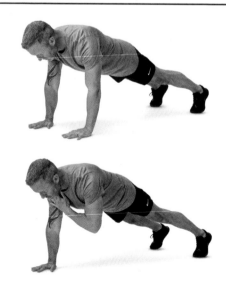

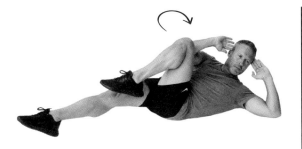

BICYCLE CRUNCHES

1 **START POSITION:** Lie on your back, with your knees bent, feet lifted, and your hands lightly touching your temples.
2 Lift your shoulders to engage the core and keep the lower back flat against the floor—not arched.
3 Twist to bring your right elbow to your left knee as you straighten your right leg. Keep alternating sides.

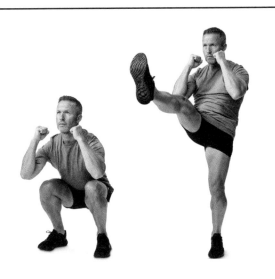

SQUAT KICKS

1 **START POSITION:** Stand with your feet shoulder-width apart and your weight in your heels.
2 Push your bottom back and bend your knees until your thighs are parallel to the ground, keeping your back straight and chest up.
3 Drive through your heels to stand back up, lift your knee, and kick one leg straight out in front of you.
4 Squeeze your glutes and keep your core tight as you return the leg to the ground and move into the next squat, kicking with the opposite leg. Repeat.

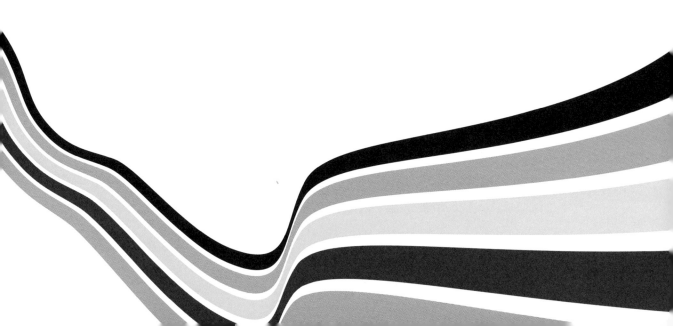

CHALLENGE 11

ONE FOR RUNNERS

- Interval runs will help build both your strength and stamina while still burning body fat.

- If you're new to running, you can start with an alternating jog/walk. Keep it simple, it's not a race, so run at your own pace—just keep going.

Warm up for 5 minutes
with a brisk walk

Run for 1 minute

Jog for 1 minute

Run for 2 minutes

Jog for 1 minute

Run for 3 minutes

Jog for 1 minute

Run for 4 minutes

Jog for 1 minute

Run for 5 minutes

Cool down for 5 minutes
with a brisk walk

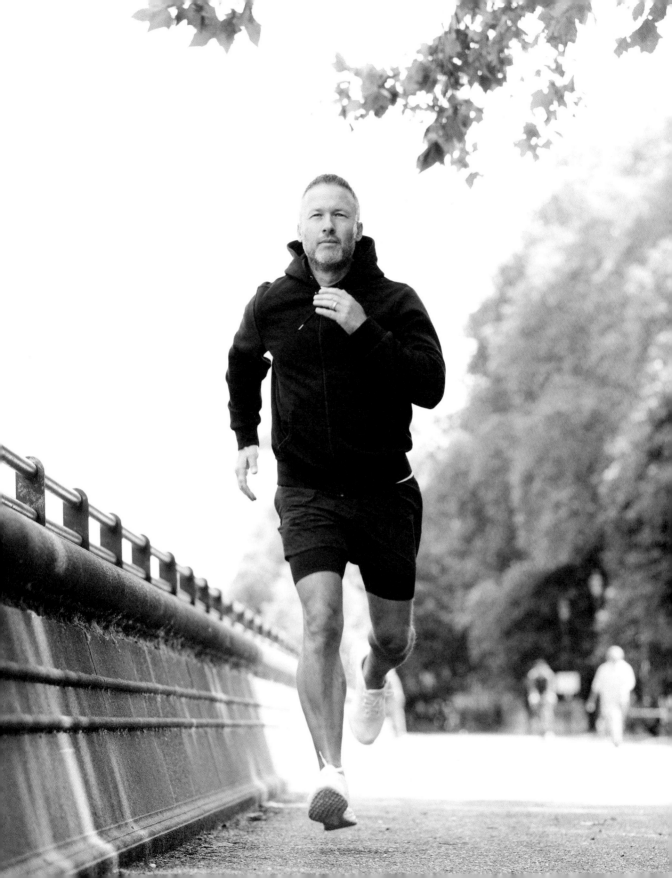

INDEX

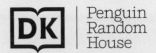

DK LONDON
Editorial Director Cara Armstrong
Senior Designer Tania Gomes
Senior Editor Alastair Laing
Production Editor David Almond
Production Controller Kariss Ainsworth
Art Director Maxine Pedliham
Publishing Director Katie Cowan

Editorial Vicki Murrell
Design Studio Nic&Lou
Photography David Cummings
Food Photography Vanessa Polignano
Stylist Dominique Eloïse Alexander

First American Edition, 2023
Published in the United States by DK Publishing
1745 Broadway, 20th Floor, New York, NY 10019

The publisher would like to thank the following for
their kind permission to reproduce their photograph:
Shutterstock.com: KADIVAR07 (Background image
used on pages 15, 18, 21, 22, 27, 167, 177, 208)
Recipe photography © Scott Harrison.
All other images © Dorling Kindersley.
For further information see www.dkimages.com

A catalog record for this book is available from
the Library of Congress.
ISBN: 978-0-7440-9460-2

DK books are available at special discounts when
purchased in bulk for sales promotions, premiums,
fund-raising, or educational use. For details, contact:
DK Publishing Special Markets at SpecialSales@dk.com.

Printed and bound in Slovakia

www.dk.com

MIX
Paper | Supporting
responsible forestry
FSC™ C018179

This book was made with Forest
Stewardship Council™ certified
paper—one small step in DK's
commitment to a sustainable future.
For more information, go to
www.dk.com/our-green-pledge.

THANK YOU

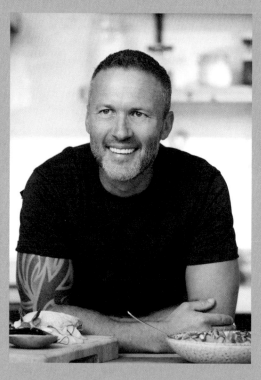

Firstly, and before I express my gratitude to my exceptional team, I want to extend a heartfelt thank you to every participant who has embraced the SPR way of life—it has been a true honor to stand by your side as you've transformed your lives in remarkable ways. You should be immensely proud of the hard work you've put into creating a healthier and happier life.

Many of you reading this will not know that every single person who works on The Six Pack Revolution has come from being a participant in the program. As it's grown exponentially over several years, I truly believe that this plays a huge part in its success, because everyone has the DNA of SPR in their blood. So, on that note, I want to acknowledge the unsung heroes behind the scenes:

My global team of motivational coaches have played an essential role in ensuring that every participant experiences the transformative magic of SPR.

My team of world-class experts (see right) are all at the pinnacle of their fields. Their knowledge and guidance have been instrumental in the evolution of the SPR program.

My beloved family—my wife and best friend, Victoria, and my children, Scarlett, Hugo, and Jasper—are my greatest blessings. The love you provide and your unwavering support mean the world to me.

My parents—for instilling in me the values of hard work and the importance of pursuing my passion.

To my management team—Sam, Annie, Sarah, and Andy—you are more than just colleagues; we are a close-knit family. I am aware of how fortunate I am to have you all by my side.

To my creative team—led by Paul "Pique" King. The quality of our collaborations is always exciting.

To Vanessa Polignano—your stunning food photography has consistently hit the mark, and it's been a pleasure collaborating with you over these years.

To Elizabeth Bullen—your ability to bring my words to life on paper is simply awesome, and it's integral to making our message resonate with our Six Pack community.

To Tom Kirby, for assisting me in creating some of these delicious meals, especially the extremely tasty vegan dishes.

To Cara, Tania, Alastair, Nikki, Vicki, and the rest of the team at Dorling Kindersley. From that first day we met, I've been blown away by your passion for what you all do and your commitment to myself and this book. May we continue to create amazing books together for years to come.

THE EXPERTS

Victoria Harrison

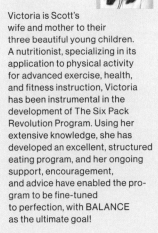

Nutritionist

Victoria is Scott's wife and mother to their three beautiful young children. A nutritionist, specializing in its application to physical activity for advanced exercise, health, and fitness instruction, Victoria has been instrumental in the development of The Six Pack Revolution Program. Using her extensive knowledge, she has developed an excellent, structured eating program, and her ongoing support, encouragement, and advice have enabled the program to be fine-tuned to perfection, with BALANCE as the ultimate goal!

Dr. Aggy York

MBChB, MRC GP

Aggy graduated from Manchester University in 2003 before going on to train in General Practice. For half of the week, she can be found at her office at the foot of the Pennines, and the rest of the week, she works as the Clinical Lead for Primary Care for the clinical commissioning group in Rochdale. Aggy considers herself a movement champion. She is an eager marathon runner, triathlete, and iron man competitor. She has helped set up a local running club and also volunteers at the local boxing club where she trains.

Dr. Miguel Guitterez

Chiropractor MChiro. S.T.R. Bio Mechanical Expert

Miguel qualified in the UK as a doctor of chiropractic medicine. He is also an expert in biomechanical dysfunction from contact sports injuries and is sought after by performers in both professional sports and the creative industries. Miguel has looked after many UK-based sports people, including bodybuilders and fighters—MMA, Shaolin monks, Kyusho Jitsu, Ryukyu Kempo, Krav Maga, Wing Chun, boxing, K-1, kickboxing, and Muay Thai. He also works tirelessly to educate all generations on the growing danger of spinal injuries in the digital age.

Dr. Joanne Farrow

Consultant Psychiatrist BM, MRCPsych, MA, MBA

Dr. Joanne Farrow is a General Adult Psychiatrist. She is a member of the Royal College of Psychiatrists and is also on the GMC Specialist Register for General Adult Psychiatry. She has also gained a master's degree in Medical Law and Ethics and a master's in Business Administration. Jo has worked in a variety of clinical settings and has experience in assessing and treating a wide range of mental health conditions and complexities, including anxiety, mood, and psychotic disorders.

Dr. Jodie Booth

Doctor of Biochemistry BSc, PhD, CSSM Dip, MISRM

Jodie has spent many years working in the human diagnostics and genetic sequencing sectors. She has always enjoyed running, cycling, and weight training, and this passion led her to become a fully qualified Soft-tissue Therapist and Personal Trainer. Now, she applies her knowledge of biochemistry to different areas of health, nutrition, and well-being.

Karen Schranz

Psychotherapist

Karen holds a bachelor's degree in Psychology, plus a master's degree in both Gestalt Psychotherapy and Human Resource Management and Training, and is a practicing psychotherapist. Karen's work focuses extensively on personal issues, such as eating and anxiety disorders, depression, bereavement, and infertility. Karen's knowledge and clear understanding of the long-term effects of eating disorders have been invaluable to the development of The Six Pack Revolution Program.

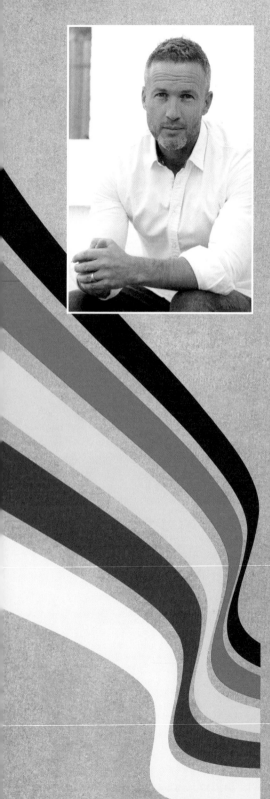

SCOTT HARRISON

Founder, The Six Pack Revolution

Scott Harrison has transformed tens of thousands of people's lives from all over the world through his incredible Six Pack Revolution Program. A qualified personal trainer, he also holds a Level 3 Psychology Diploma, plus he's a black-belt karate instructor (who has competed at a national level), a proud dad to three beautiful children, and a loving husband, too.

Scott is a major advocate for the immeasurable benefits of health and fitness, and his program is not only training celebrities and motivating everyone, of all ages, to transform their physical and mental health but also alleviating so many debilitating illnesses and conditions. There is nothing Scott enjoys more than spreading the SPR magic worldwide. He is very proud of the way The Six Pack Revolution has benefited the lives of so many and hopes it will continue to do so for many years to come.

FINAL WORD

It has been a pleasure to share my passion with you in this book, and I hope that it has given you a blueprint so that you can also experience a transformative journey with the Six Pack Revolution Program. Every page has been written with love to give you the knowledge and self-belief that you need to move forward and become a better you!

I hope that you have found the book rewarding, and I'd love to hear from you about how you are doing. Please feel free to post on our social media pages (TikTok, Instagram, Facebook: @thesixpackrevolution; Twitter: @6packrevolution) about any progress you have made, or to comment on your favorite recipes, or anything else for that matter.

I'd like to finish by extending a heartfelt thank you to everyone, past and present, who has contributed to The Six Pack Revolution in any way, shape, or form. Let's continue to uplift, inspire, and focus on self-love and respect for each other. When we have a healthy body and mind, it makes it so much easier to find the positives in life.

Wishing you all the love and luck in the world.

Much love

Scotty x